"*The Mind's Own Physician* is a journey of understanding, in which an integrative dialogue unfolds between the spiritual leaders of contemplative meditation and scientists at the forefront of mind-body medicine. This transformative conversation provides valuable insight into how meditative practices can balance the mind with effects on the body, as well as, potential benefits for human health. This blending of contemplative traditions with Western science opens a mindful awareness that has the empowering capacity to fully engage people in their health, and more broadly, in the well-being of our societies."

—Michael R. Irwin, MD, Cousins Professor of Psychiatry and Biobehavioral Sciences, David Geffen School of Medicine, University of California, Los Angeles

"*The Mind's Own Physician* offers us a precious portal into the seminal conversations that gave birth to the nascent field of contemplative neuroscience. The issues digested, debated, and ignited in its pages will serve as a road map and inspiration for my students and their students over the coming decades."

—Amishi P. Jha, PhD, contemplative neuroscientist, Associate Professor of Psychology, University of Miami

"If you want to see how to build bridges between the deepest wisdom of the heart and the highest standards of contemporary neuroscience, look no further. This series of meetings between His Holiness the Dalai Lama and Western scientists and meditation teachers will prove to be epoch-changing, and this book shows why. Here, you will find interior and exterior empiricism in exquisite dialogue. Drink it all in. The brilliance of the participants shines through on every page."

—Mark Williams, PhD, Professor of Clinical Psychology, University of Oxford, Director, Oxford Mindfulness Centre

"Can meditation improve your health? This question is just the starting point for a series of innovative exchanges across different ways of knowing among first-ranked clinicians, scientists, Buddhist teachers, and the Dalai Lama. Thoughtful, rigorous, and surprising by turns, this dialogue reminds all of us who care about the effects of the mind on health just how much more thinking remains to be done."

—Anne Harrington, PhD, Professor of the History of Science, Harvard University, author of *The Cure Within*

"Our thoughts can seem too real, giving our imaginings about tomorrow the power to create chronic stress and unhealthy changes in our bodies. Our sense of self can seem too fixed, creating a cage where our habitual worries can run in depressing circles. In the moment that we recognize our thoughts as thoughts and our habits as habits, new and liberating possibilities emerge for the way we live our lives. Contemplative traditions such as Buddhism have long seen the transformative power of that simple moment of recognition, and more recently, clinicians in various domains have discovered the potential that this contemplative insight offers for the treatment of chronic stress, depression, and other especially modern maladies. Yet the potential of interventions based on contemplative approaches has only begun to emerge. The full realization of that potential requires a careful, critical, and honest dialogue among contemplatives and scientists so as to allow research and clinical practices to develop effectively. This remarkable book provides a fresh and clear record of such a dialogue. Informative and highly accessible, *The Mind's Own Physician* is a groundbreaking moment in the development of contemplative science."

—John D. Dunne, Associate Professor of Religion, Emory University

"A must-read for anyone interested in understanding how Buddhist contemplative traditions and Western scientific traditions can work together to uncover the complexities of the human mind. Mind and Life has done it again: engaged a group of distinguished contemplative scholars, clinicians, and scientists in a lively, productive, and inspiring dialogue with His Holiness the Dalai Lama that furthers our understanding of meditation and its potential to heal."

—Jeanne Tsai, Associate Professor of Psychology, Stanford University, Director, Stanford Culture and Emotion Laboratory

"This book marks a milestone in the emerging field of contemplative sciences. With this book, you can relive a seminal 2005 Mind and Life conference that brought together world-famous neuroscientists, clinicians, and contemplative scholars in a dialogue with His Holiness the Dalai Lama. This groundbreaking work explores the development of scientifically based tools and programs aimed at creating more balanced and healthy lives. How does stress evolve? What does it do to our minds and bodies? How can we use ancient mindfulness and meditative practices in our everyday, modern lives and also in clinical settings to reduce stress and cultivate healthier minds? This book is a must for everyone who is interested in making this world a more human place."

—Tania Singer, PhD, Director, Department of Social Neuroscience, Max Planck Institute for Human Cognitive and Brain Sciences, Leipzig, Germany

"Jon Kabat-Zinn and Richard Davidson bring together an internationally acclaimed cast of neuroscientists and scholars for a stimulating dialogue with the Dalai Lama. They weave a rich tapestry of information on how meditation can be useful for a wide variety of conditions, ranging from depression and stress to anxiety and psoriasis. In easy-to-understand, conversational style, the experts lay out how the mind's powerful healing effects can be harnessed in ways that are becoming increasingly illuminated by scientific discoveries."

—Stuart J. Eisendrath, MD, Professor of Psychiatry, University of California, San Francisco, Director of the UCSF Depression Center

"It is most befitting that this wonderful book, composed from Mind and Life dialogues with His Holiness the Dalai Lama, would appear after the tenth anniversary of the September 11, 2001 tragedy. Accompanied by greatly increasing psychophysiological stress, anxiety, and depression, the post-9/11 decade has yielded an auspicious upsurge of rigorous scientific and clinical research on mindfulness meditation and other systematic methods of mental training that may help transcend the pain and suffering caused by such harmful afflictions. *The Mind's Own Physician* highlights these exciting advances through a series of insightful discussions between His Holiness and a diverse group of stellar contemplative scholars, scientists, and physicians who are leaders in the field of integrative mind-body-brain medicine. Everyone who wishes to cultivate a sound body and sane, healthy mind in these turbulent times will welcome the publication of these inspiring conversations."

—David E. Meyer, PhD, Clyde H. Coombs, and J. E. Keith Smith Professor of Mathematical Psychology and Cognitive Science, University of Michigan

"A fascinating book exploring two contrasting views of the human mind. The scholarly discussions between His Holiness and leading scientists provide deep insights into how ancient Buddhist teachings and modern science can inform each other, and potentially transform Western clinical practices."

—Sara Lazar, PhD, Associate in Psychology, Psychiatric Neuroscience Research Program, Massachusetts General Hospital, Instructor of Psychiatry, Harvard Medical School

"*The Mind's Own Physician* brings you straight into the heart of a remarkable interchange between His Holiness the Dalai Lama, renowned contemplative teachers from Buddhist and Christian traditions, and world leaders in neuroscience, psychiatry, stress physiology, and clinical medicine. Jon Kabat-Zinn and Richard Davidson guide the reader through an authentic chronicle of a landmark meeting of extraordinary minds as it unfolds through a series of crystalline presentations and probing dialogues about the nature of mind, meditation, and brain function. These dialogues provide the foundation for discussion on the biological effects of chronic stress, treatment and relapse prevention in depression, and the historical and evolutionary roots of Western medicine's struggle to understand and care for the whole person. The highly accessible and rich treatment of each of these areas is fascinating to read. The constant presence of His Holiness the Dalai Lama's deeply engaged attention, teaching, and critical ear reverberates throughout. The participants' common commitment to fostering the conditions necessary for human flourishing through intercultural and interdisciplinary inquiry is truly inspiring. In capturing this arc of information and intent, *The Mind's Own Physician* becomes an essential treatment of one of the most hopeful directions in thought alive today: the human capacity to ease our suffering through introspective insight and our growing scientific investigation into how this may occur."

—Clifford Saron, PhD, Associate Research Scientist, University of California, Davis Center for Mind and Brain

"It is extremely exciting to read what emerges from the dialogues between the leading experts in the scientific investigation of contemplative practice who present their excellent scientific work and the profound wisdom of contemplative teachers. This is a wonderful book that takes us right into the heart of these inspiring and engaging conversations by exploring profound and essential questions about how we can enhance human potential by cultivating positive human qualities."

—Britta Hölzel, PhD, Research Fellow, Massachusetts General Hospital, Harvard Medical School, and Bender Institute of Neuroimaging, Giessen University, Germany

"*The Mind's Own Physician* is a remarkable accomplishment. It tells the compelling story of how the scientific study of meditation has created a new way of understanding the relationship between body and mind and between science and spirituality. Edited by Jon Kabat-Zinn and Richard Davidson, two individuals who have almost single-handedly brought mindfulness into Western culture, it documents a dialogue between the Dalai Lama and a gathering of researchers, scholars, and clinicians who are blazing new pathways in the science of meditation. The discussion highlights how the neuroscience of meditation is enriching our understanding of human potential. This is a deeply hopeful book. It details how many of the qualities most urgently needed in our world today can be intentionally cultivated in practical, concrete ways that make a real difference. Compassion, wisdom, insight, and emotional balance are not lucky accidents; they are biological capabilities that can be strengthened. *The Mind's Own Physician* is essential reading for anyone who wants to learn about the ancient tradition of meditation, the promise that it holds for our time, and the essential goodness of the human spirit."

> —Michael J. Baime, MD, Clinical Associate Professor of Medicine, Perelman School of Medicine, University of Pennsylvania, Founder and Director, Penn Program for Mindfulness

"Besides engaging easily with the contemplative, clinical, and scientific contributions to this volume, the reader experiences the remarkable interaction of contributors from diverse traditions. Common assumptions become apparent, constructs in one discipline spark insights in another, broad inter-disciplinary understandings subsume disciplinary understandings. Over the course of the exchange, it becomes apparent that a new culture is emerging with the potential to fundamentally reshape how we understand ourselves and interact with one another."

> —Lawrence W. Barsalou, PhD, Samuel Candler Dobbs Professor of Psychology, Emory University

"*The Mind's Own Physician* lets us eavesdrop on a fascinating conversation at the frontier of science and spirituality, medicine and meditation. Anyone who cares about well-being and health will find both news and wisdom here."

> —Daniel Goleman, PhD, author of *The Brain and Emotional Intelligence*

MIND AND LIFE PUBLICATIONS

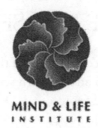

MIND & LIFE
INSTITUTE

In addition to *The Mind's Own Physician*, the Mind and Life Institute has published several books and DVD sets that explore the dialogues between His Holiness the Dalai Lama and leading scientists.

MIND AND LIFE BOOKS

- *Gentle Bridges: Conversations with the Dalai Lama on the Sciences of Mind* (1987)

- *Consciousness at the Crossroads: Conversations with the Dalai Lama on Brain Science and Buddhism* (1989)

- *Healing Emotions: Conversations with the Dalai Lama on Mindfulness, Emotions, and Health* (1990)

- *Visions of Compassion: Western Scientists and Tibetan Buddhists Examine Human Nature* (1995)

- *Sleeping, Dreaming, and Dying: An Exploration of Consciousness with the Dalai Lama* (1992)

- *The New Physics and Cosmology: Dialogues with the Dalai Lama* (1997)

- *Destructive Emotions: A Scientific Dialogue with the Dalai Lama* (2000)

- *Mind and Life: Discussions with the Dalai Lama on the Nature of Reality* (2002)

- *The Dalai Lama at MIT* (2003)
- *Train Your Mind, Change Your Brain* (2004)

MIND AND LIFE DVD SETS

The following DVD sets are compilations of the actual dialogues between His Holiness the Dalai Lama and Western scientists. DVD sets are available online at www.mindandlife.org.

- *Investigating the Mind* (2003)
- *The Science and Clinical Applications of Meditation* (2005)
- *The Science of a Compassionate Life* (2006)
- *Educating World Citizens for the 21st Century* (2009)
- *Altruism and Compassion in Economic Systems* (2010)

MIND AND LIFE ONLINE VIDEO

- *The Scientific Study of Contemplative Practice on Human Biology and Behaviour* (2010), available free online at www.mindandlife.org.

THE MIND'S OWN PHYSICIAN

A SCIENTIFIC DIALOGUE *with*
the DALAI LAMA *on the* HEALING
POWER *of* MEDITATION

EDITED BY JON KABAT-ZINN, PHD
& RICHARD J. DAVIDSON, PHD
WITH ZARA HOUSHMAND

MIND & LIFE INSTITUTE
NEW HARBINGER PUBLICATIONS, INC.

Distributed in Canada by Raincoast Books

Copyright © 2011 by Jon Kabat-Zinn and Richard J. Davidson
        New Harbinger Publications, Inc.
        5674 Shattuck Avenue
        Oakland, CA 94609
        www.newharbinger.com

Cover design by Amy Shoup; Text design by Michele Waters-Kermes;
Acquired by Catharine Meyers; Edited by Jasmine Star

Library of Congress Cataloging-in-Publication Data

The mind's own physician : a scientific dialogue with the Dalai Lama on the healing power of meditation / edited by Jon Kabat-Zinn and Richard J. Davidson with Zara Houshmand.
    p. cm.
  Includes bibliographical references and index.
  ISBN 978-1-57224-968-4 (pbk.) -- ISBN 978-1-57224-969-1 (pdf e-book)
  1. Buddhism--Psychology. 2. Meditation--Buddhism. 3. Mental healing. 4. Spiritual healing. 5. Brain--Psychophysiology. I. Bstan-'dzin-rgya-mtsho, Dalai Lama XIV, 1935- II. Kabat-Zinn, Jon. III. Davidson, Richard J. IV. Houshmand, Zara.
  BQ4570.P76M56 2012
  294.3'36150--dc23

                2011031863

13   12   11

10   9   8   7   6   5   4   3   2   1

First printing

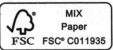

CONTENTS

Introduction

A Confluence of Streams and a Flowering of Possibilities

An extraordinary confluence of epistemologies, or different ways of knowing, is unfolding in the present era. Not too long ago, Gary Snyder, poet, essayist, and naturalist, evoked the image of glaciers slowly but inexorably merging, while still maintaining some evidence of their origins in the streaks they display: "We stand on the lateral moraine of the glacier eased along by Newton and Descartes. The revivified Goddess Gaia glacier is coming down another valley, from our distant pagan past, and another arm of ice is sliding in from another angle: the no-nonsense meditation view of Buddhism with its emphasis on compassion and insight in an empty universe."[1]

Yet now we know, a mere two decades later, that the earth's glaciers are literally, not metaphorically, on a rapid trajectory toward disappearing altogether. Perhaps the metaphor was fated to become inadequate, given the unprecedented rate of change humanity is generating on this earth, the consequences of which we are just waking up to. It may be more apt at this point in history to speak of the convergence of epistemologies and cultures as streams flowing rapidly together, rather than as glaciers. This more liquid and turbulent metaphor speaks to the many different traditions, disciplines, perspectives, and technologies that are currently encountering each other in unpredictable ways. Time will tell. And it will not be a long time, given the rate at which things are unfolding.

The specific convergence we are referring to here, dead-on explicit in Snyder's musing, is that of science with the contemplative traditions, and the meditative traditions in particular. These are indeed different epistemologies—different ways of investigating, explaining, and ultimately shaping human experience and our relationship to the larger world we find ourselves embedded in. Never before have modern science and the contemplative traditions come together to inform each other as they are now, as witnessed by this volume and others on the Mind and Life Dialogues, documenting aspects of an even larger admixing taking place in this era. Both are ancient and venerable traditions. Both have their own recognized lineages, along with noteworthy milestones that illuminate with precision and some degree of authority the hard-won findings of the systematic and disciplined investigations of reality by people who cared and care deeply to understand, and who left a trail for others by documenting their experience and findings with maximal precision and rigor, according to specific methodologies and hypotheses nurtured by powerful motivations akin, ultimately, to love.

In the case of science, the reality in question, up to now, has been primarily outer directed: concern for the nature of nature and our place in it, for the essence of reality and the laws governing phenomena, and more oriented toward understanding the observed than the observer. To this end, methods and instruments have evolved and are continually evolving to accurately probe the nature of matter and energy, its manifestations from elementary particles to the most highly complex assemblies of matter in the known-by-us universe, namely ourselves, and the undeniable sentience that mysteriously emerges within complex living systems and particularly our species—*Homo sapiens sapiens*—and shapes our societies and cultures.

In the case of the contemplative traditions, the vector of inquiry and investigation up to now has been primarily inward directed, probing the domain of the mind. Yet until recently, interior experience was dismissed in some academic circles as merely "subjective," as opposed to "objective." Now it is getting a second look as an essential and valid phenomenological dimension of human experience and knowing. This more balanced view, reconfigured as first-person experience, is thanks in large measure to

Francisco Varela. Since nothing in science to date actually explains the nature of our interior experience,[2] it seems prudent to at least entertain the possibility that a systematic investigation of inner experience from the first-person perspective has its own valid parameters as an epistemology, and has the potential (especially coupled with third-person methodologies) to contribute profoundly to a balanced and collaborative investigation of what we call the mind and human experience, including the dilemmas of suffering, greed, aggression, delusion, and ignorance, the tyranny and dangers inherent in Socrates's "unexamined life"—the mind that, contrary to the appellation *Homo sapiens sapiens*, does not know itself. This is the very much alive and relevant arena of the contemplative traditions, what might be called their "laboratory domain."

Of course, it is a heuristic conceit and a gross generalization to speak of science as outer directed and the meditative traditions as inner directed. Many fields within science are concerned with studying the nature of mental phenomena, and contemplative wisdom does not make a distinction between outer and inner, recognizing that they are different aspects of a deeper, non-dual wholeness, and that the ultimate realization of any introspective process manifests in how one lives one's life. Nevertheless, there has been at least the appearance of a predominantly outer-directed mind-set and mode of investigation on the part of science and an inward investigation on the part of the meditative traditions. The Mind and Life Dialogues are contributing to the examination and breaking down of such categories and a cross-fertilization of ways of knowing and viable research endeavors at the interfaces of these larger trends.[3]

A BRIEF HISTORY

In this volume, the convergence of science and the contemplative traditions is represented by the coming together of highly regarded and experienced practitioners in both worlds to meet in conversation on the topic "The Science and Clinical Applications of Meditation." A gathering of this scope and magnitude would have been unthinkable ten or fifteen years ago. Yet it came to pass in 2005, arising from an earlier and equally unthinkable public meeting held at MIT,[4] and from a stream of smaller invitational meetings that have taken place since 1987 under the auspices of the Mind and Life Institute and with the abiding interest and enthusiastic engagement of His Holiness the Dalai Lama.

It is widely known that the Dalai Lama has had a lifelong passion for science and its potential, with all its attendant limits, for contributing to a deep understanding of natural phenomena and an elucidation of the nature of things. As a consequence, he has been engaging scientists both privately and publicly his entire life. At first, the Mind and Life meetings took place in private, usually at the Dalai Lama's residence in Dharamsala, India. They were conceived as a kind of tutorial for His Holiness to familiarize himself with various domains of science that he was particularly interested in but had never had the occasion to study as part of his traditional education as a Buddhist monk, especially given his unique life situation from the age of two as the recognized incarnation of the previous Dalai Lama, and thus the titular leader of all Tibetan Buddhists as well as the leader of the Tibetan people. However, in the early Mind and Life meetings, it rapidly became clear that His Holiness's grasp of the concepts and experiments being described to him was that of a natural-born scientist. He was often out ahead of the explanations, asking cogent questions and anticipating the next experiments. Moreover, it quickly became evident that the scientists involved were at least as profoundly affected by this modest Buddhist monk as he was by them.

Thus, the Mind and Life Dialogues became an ongoing mutual exploration of some of the most profound questions facing humanity in terms of science, ethics, and morality, such as the nature of mind, the nature of the universe and our place in it, the nature of reality, and the potential for the healing and transformation of afflictive emotions into more positive mental states, leading to greater health, harmony, happiness, and possibly both inner and outer peace. Over the years, these dialogues have included psychologists and neuroscientists, physicians and philosophers, physicists, molecular biologists, and educators, and also contemplatives and monastics from various Buddhist lineages as well as other spiritual traditions. Increasingly, more Tibetan monks and nuns have joined as observers and students of these dialogues as a result of His Holiness's efforts to promote a greater exposure to the modern scientific worldview within the monastic community. Each meeting has resulted in a book describing the proceedings and capturing, in large measure and each in its own unique way, the excitement and power of open minds in true dialogue, together exploring fundamental questions of potentially profound import to the modern world. (For a listing of all the Mind and Life books, see the beginning of the book or www.mindandlife.org/publications.)

In the 2000 meeting, described in the book *Destructive Emotions*,[5] His Holiness urged participants to find innovative ways to make the meditative practices being elucidated as effective in regulating difficult emotions more accessible in wholly secular contexts, since their essence is grounded in universal aspects of the human mind and heart, and thus their potential benefits are not at all limited to adherents of Buddhism. Such universalized approaches to the potential benefits of meditative practices are all the more important and urgent given the prevalence of depression, anxiety, and post-traumatic stress disorder, as well as the high levels of stress and violence, that characterize our modern age.

Around the same time, the Dalai Lama also urged the leadership of the Mind and Life Institute to organize shorter public dialogues that more students, scientists, and scholars could attend, in addition to the five-day more private meetings that had been the traditional format in Dharamsala. The idea was that this would allow more people to participate directly, through their physical presence, in the energies of these collective inquiries, and thus perhaps be inspired to pursue new lines of research and societal applications based on what was emerging from these conversations.

The first public dialogue, Mind and Life XI, held September 13 and 14, 2003, at MIT, was cosponsored by the McGovern Institute for Brain Research at MIT. It was entitled "Investigating the Mind: Exchanges between Buddhism and Biobehavioral Science" and featured a range of neuroscientists, psychologists, and scholars. It was documented in the book *The Dalai Lama at MIT*, edited by Anne Harrington and Arthur Zajonc.[6] The very fact that the conference took place at MIT was itself historic, a major and early public acknowledgment of the confluence of these diverse ways of investigating the mind and the world. The level of engagement in the dialogue and the reflections of participants a year after it took place give the interested reader a rich and enduring tapestry of information, attitudinal perspectives, and insights from the participants about both the value and the limitations—and even the frustrations—of such attempts at understanding and collaboration across what can easily seem like an unbridgeable chasm between vastly different cultures and worldviews.

THE CONTEXT OF THE 2005 MEETING: MIND AND LIFE XIII

After the MIT meeting, which focused primarily on basic research questions in the specific disciplines of attention and cognitive control, emotion, and mental imagery, and how these activities are expressed and regulated in the brain, it was decided that the next public meeting (Mind and Life XIII, to be held in 2005) should address the remarkable rise in clinical applications of meditation within Western medicine and psychology, and the clinical and basic science undergirding these developments. The board of the Mind and Life Institute, which includes the editors of the present volume, based this decision in part on the preponderance of questions from the MIT audience concerning practical applications of meditation practices to their personal situations and, more generally, to health-related concerns. Unfortunately, the presenters could not address such questions, as they were not germane to the topic of the 2003 meeting. But the volume of that kind of question did indicate a widespread interest in applications of meditative practices in both medicine and personal life, prompting us to take notice and respond.

This book documents that second, equally historic and groundbreaking public meeting between His Holiness and scientists: Mind and Life XIII, "The Science and Clinical Applications of Meditation." Its title, *The Mind's Own Physician*, points to the self-healing nature of the human organism and the potential of systematic mental training to optimize the dynamical balance that is what is meant by the term "health" on multiple levels, including the cognitive, emotional, visceral, somatic, relational, and transcendent. Much of the evidence supporting that potential was presented at this meeting.

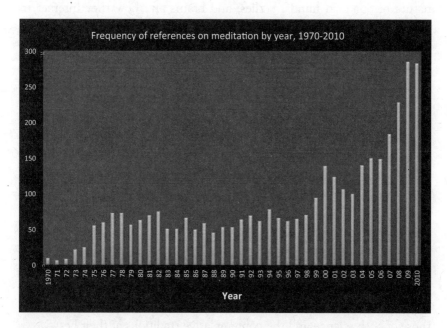

Figure 1. Results obtained from a search of the term "meditation" in the abstract and key words of the ISI Web of Knowledge database on February 5, 2011. The search was limited to publications with English language abstracts. Figure prepared by David S. Black, Institute for Prevention Research, Keck School of Medicine, University of Southern California.

Figure 1 shows the rise in the number of papers on meditation published in the medical and scientific literature between 1970 and 2010. Indeed, this curve and the curve for mindfulness alone[7] seem to be increasing exponentially at this juncture. Funding for meditation research has increased at a similar rate. This phenomenon was already well under way at the time of Mind and Life XIII, in 2005. It is dramatic evidence of the speed at which modern science is now converging with meditative practices from the contemplative traditions, at this time primarily Buddhism. (More recently, Mind and Life XXII, held in New Delhi, India, in November 2010, expanded the dialogue to include yoga and meditative practices from other traditions.)

The increase in meditation research in recent decades is perhaps only one manifestation of a broadly distributive, collaborative, and highly intentional investigation, through multiple complementary lenses, of the nature of our own minds, bodies, and brains and how they interact to influence health and disease, well-being and suffering, happiness and depression, and, ultimately, our basic humanity. Its promise and import seem to lie in examining and understanding our potential for ongoing development as conscious and compassionate beings—our capacity to grow into what is deepest and best in ourselves both as individuals and as a species—perhaps in time to avert some of the present and potentially impending disasters we face as a result of being a precocious species on a limited and fragile planet.

The Latin *Homo sapiens sapiens* means, literally, the species that knows and knows that it knows. The species name itself captures our core capacity for awareness and meta-awareness. Perhaps it is time for us to live our way into this potential of ours as a species before it is too late. And since meditation has everything to do with awareness and attention and their refinement through practice, this itself is a major nexus of serendipitous convergence from which humanity may ultimately benefit by drawing upon all of its various wisdom traditions and methodologies, including those of both science and the contemplative traditions at their best.

The 2003 meeting at MIT was held at Kresge Auditorium, filled to capacity with twelve hundred people. Given the huge interest in the clinical applications of meditation, we felt it was important to hold the second public meeting in an even larger venue so that more people could participate through their presence and their deep listening, and through the spontaneous conversations that tend to arise within such a highly motivated audience outside the formal sessions. Perhaps this is one of the most important and creative functions of any conference, providing informal and unstructured opportunities for communication, within which much of the ongoing creative impact occurs, setting the stage for and often catalyzing the next generation of ideas and collaborations.

Originally, it was hoped that the National Institutes of Health (NIH) would cosponsor the meeting and host it at its campus in Bethesda, especially since it had already held a daylong symposium in March of 2004 on the subject "Mindfulness Meditation and Health," which had been very well attended and engendered a great deal of enthusiasm. However, that option proved to be too complicated for numerous reasons, so the meeting was held from November 8-10, 2005, in downtown Washington, DC, at Constitution Hall, which holds over three thousand people. It was cosponsored by the Johns Hopkins University School of Medicine and Georgetown University Medical Center.

The very fact that MIT, and then Johns Hopkins and Georgetown Universities aligned themselves with a world-renowned spiritual leader of the Dalai Lama's stature in a dialogue of this kind is itself extraordinary, and an indicator of the degree to which the convergence of streams and worldviews is taking place. At the MIT meeting, Eric Lander opined that perhaps MIT and the McGovern Institute for Brain Research were secure enough in their scientific reputations to "not fear pushing the envelope a bit" in terms of the risks, real and imagined, of engaging in such a cross-cultural dialogue.[8] It is evidence that the world is indeed changing and growing into a recognition that we humans probably need to understand ourselves as a species from multiple perspectives in order to realize our full potential. In a similar vein, just prior to the 2005 Mind and Life Dialogue at Constitution Hall, the Dalai Lama gave a keynote address to the annual meeting of the Society for Neuroscience, which happened to be holding its meeting in Washington that same week. Over twenty-five thousand neuroscientists attended the lecture. This was a similarly unprecedented event for a scientific congress.

The Presenters

The presenters, panelists, and session moderators for this event were selected on the basis of their expertise and leadership in science, medicine, and the meditative traditions, and for their remarkable breadth of training and experience as individuals at the interfaces of different disciplines and epistemologies. Richard Davidson and Jon Kabat-Zinn, the co-organizers of the meeting, guided the selection with input from the Mind and Life board of directors and community.

THE CONTEMPLATIVE PARTICIPANTS

On the contemplative side, His Holiness the Dalai Lama was the catalyst for the meeting and a critical participant in all sessions, except for the interlude between sessions 3 and 4, as were his interpreters, Thupten Jinpa, PhD, and Alan Wallace, PhD. During the interlude on the second day,

Alan also gave a lunchtime talk establishing a broad context for understanding meditation from the contemplative perspective. Jinpa was a monk for many years before returning to lay life as a husband, father, and exponent of translating important Tibetan texts into modern languages. After leaving the monkhood, he received his PhD from Cambridge University in religious studies. Alan Wallace was also a monk for many years and a student of His Holiness, as well as many other Tibetan Buddhist teachers. He trained in physics and philosophy and has written prolifically on science, Buddhism, and Buddhist meditation practices. He received his PhD from Stanford University in religious studies.

Father Thomas Keating contributed his good nature and his experience and perspective from the Christian monastic Cistercian Order and as a principal in pioneering the development of the modern movement of centering prayer. Ajahn Amaro represented the Theravada Thai forest monastic tradition, and Matthieu Ricard (along with His Holiness and his translators) represented the Tibetan Buddhist monastic tradition. Interestingly, both Ajahn Amaro and Matthieu had an early foundation in Western science, Ajahn Amaro receiving a BS in psychology and physiology from the University of London, and Matthieu a PhD in cellular genetics from the Pasteur Institute with Nobel laureate François Jacob.

Also contributing to the dialogue from the contemplative side were Sharon Salzberg, representing the vipassana tradition in the West, who also guided the audience in a meditation on loving-kindness; Jan Chozen Bays, MD, both a Zen roshi and a pediatrician with expertise in child abuse and addictions; Joan Halifax, PhD, also a Zen roshi with a wide background in medical anthropology and psychology; and Jack Kornfield, PhD, formerly a monk in the Thai forest tradition and a vipassana teacher and psychologist.

From even this cursory synopsis, it is apparent how varied and multifaceted the backgrounds and meditative training of this group of contemplatives have been. It could be said that each one, through his or her unique life trajectory and commitments, represents the larger confluence of streams that the meeting itself embodied. All were well equipped to engage in the collective inquiry and dialogue, present their own perspectives on the subject at hand, and consider critically the various lines of evidence and argument presented by the scientists.

THE SCIENTIFIC PARTICIPANTS

On the science side, we invited a range of presenters and panelists who could help us explore the potential implications of some of the most recent basic science that provides a framework for understanding the possible mechanisms through which meditation might exert its various effects. We also looked to these participants to help us examine clinical research findings on the applications of meditation for specific physical and psychiatric illnesses.

Robert Sapolsky, PhD, of Stanford University, was there to discuss his pioneering work on stress and disease at the neuronal and gene expression levels. Wolf Singer, MD, PhD, of the Max Planck Institute for Brain Research in Frankfurt, presented his work on distributive cortical processing of percepts and the phenomenon of synchronization of gamma waves in the brain, and their possible relationship to meditative practices and states of mind. Zindel Segal, PhD, from the Centre for Addiction and Mental Health at the University of Toronto and one of the founders of mindfulness-based cognitive therapy, presented on preventing relapse in people with a history of major depressive disorder. Helen Mayberg, MD, of the Emory University School of Medicine, whose work with neuroimaging has elucidated neural pathways that may play a role in major depression, addressed a variety of treatment approaches, from medications and cognitive behavioral therapy to direct modulation of specific circuits using deep-brain stimulation. John Sheridan, PhD, from Ohio State University, brought expertise on the effects of stress on the hypothalamic-pituitary-adrenal axis, as well as interactions between brain, body, behavior, and the immune system. Margaret Kemeny, PhD, of the University of California, San Francisco, offered her perspective on possible links between psychosocial factors, the immune system, and health and illness. Esther Sternberg, MD, of the NIH, provided her expertise on mechanisms of neuroimmune modulation and mind/body interactions in relationship to stress, disease, and health.

Other participants from the science side included John Teasdale, PhD, an expert on the modeling of information-based pathways for emotional expression in the brain and central nervous system, and a cofounder of mindfulness-based cognitive therapy for depression (with Zindel Segal and Mark Williams). At the time of the meeting, John had retired from Cambridge University, MRC Cognition and Brain Sciences Unit, and was in training as a meditation teacher in the vipassana tradition. We were also joined by David Sheps, MD, of the Emory University School of Medicine, an expert on mental stress–induced ischemia in cardiovascular disease and mortality, and at the time editor in chief of the journal *Psychosomatic Medicine*; biochemist Bennett Shapiro, MD, former vice president of Merck Research Laboratories, an expert in the molecular regulation of cellular behavior, and a member of the board of the Mind and Life Institute; and Ralph Snyderman, MD, chancellor emeritus of the Duke University School of Medicine, a rheumatologist by training and a leading figure in health care reform and integrative medicine.

The scientific complement of our meeting included its co-convenors and the editors of this volume, Jon Kabat-Zinn, PhD, the developer of mindfulness-based stress reduction from the University of Massachusetts Medical School, and Richard J. Davidson, PhD, of the University of Wisconsin, a founder of the field of affective neuroscience and the nascent field of contemplative neuroscience, both also board members of the Mind and Life Institute.

THE STATE OF THE SCIENCE: 2005 TO 2011

The closing chapter of this book will summarize some of the exciting new developments that have taken place in the science and clinical applications of meditation in the intervening years. In 2005, the field was still young. Six years later, we could say that that is still very much the case. Yet so much more work is now being done in the field as meditation in general and mindfulness-based interventions specifically become recognized lines of research and authentic career-building trajectories for young clinicians and basic scientists. Because of the rate at which the field is advancing (illustrated by figure 1), almost twice as many papers were published in 2010 as in 2005. Thus, the 2005 meeting both took a reading of the status of the field at that time and helped define some of the promise that seems to have propelled it forward.

Since the time of the meeting, a new professional journal called *Mindfulness* has appeared (2010), as well as a website that offers a comprehensive listing of all research papers on mindfulness, including a monthly bulletin with updated listings (*Mindfulness Research Monthly*; http.mindfulexperience.org/newsletter.php). Moreover, several premier journals have devoted either special issues or special sections to mindfulness (for example, *Emotion* in 2010,[9] *Journal of Clinical Psychology* in 2009,[10] and *Journal of Cognitive Psychotherapy* in 2009[11]), and it is likely that more are in the pipeline. Of considerable note is that one of the professional journals that has devoted a special issue to the topic of mindfulness isn't a scientific publication at all but a journal dedicated primarily to Buddhist scholarship in the modern context: *Contemporary Buddhism*. The journal's editor in chief invited Mark Williams of Oxford University and Jon Kabat-Zinn of the University of Massachusetts Medical School to be guest editors of the issue, published in July of 2011,[12] which is structured explicitly to encourage a cross-discipline conversation among Buddhist scholars, clinicians, and scientists on topics related to mindfulness as it moves increasingly into mainstream secular settings and applications. Among other topics, it addresses the question of definitions of mindfulness and issues related to the fidelity of modern mindfulness-based interventions to the original teachings as documented in early Buddhist texts and those of later schools as Buddhism spread from India and Southeast Asia into China, Tibet, Korea, and Japan over the first millennium following the Buddha's death. Such an improbable scholarly conversation across widely divergent disciplines is highly indicative of the degree to which the confluence of streams has already occurred, and speaks to its multidirectional nature.

A COZY SETTING

At Mind and Life XIII, in Washington, DC, our intention was to replicate onstage, to whatever degree possible given the large audience, the cozy and friendly environment of the private meetings that take place in His Holiness's compound in McLeod Ganj, Upper Dharamsala, India, a lovely hill station town perched under the towering snowcapped foothills of the Himalayas.

Although private, those meetings always include a number of observers in addition to the presenters. Some are contemplatives, including monastics enrolled in a program called the Science for Monks project.

Others include family members of the presenters, supporters and staff of the Mind and Life Institute, His Holiness's personal guests, and the occasional journalist.

The physical arrangement is always the same. His Holiness sits, usually cross-legged, in a big chair in the center, with the moderator and the various presenters and panelists for that session to his right and left around a low table. Immediately on his left are his two translators, so they can huddle together with His Holiness when the need to consult about the meaning of a particular term or the drift of an argument requires a temporary halt to the proceedings. His Holiness sometimes speaks in English and sometimes in Tibetan. Sometimes he begins in one language and transitions to the other. His English is very good, and he can follow complex scientific arguments if the presenter avoids the jargon that specialists can so easily fall into. Often he interrupts to ask the presenter a question or confer with his translators. When he chooses to speak in Tibetan, Thupten Jinpa then conveys in English what he said. (In this book, the translated speeches are represented as His Holiness's own words, without noting Thupten Jinpa's role except where he contributes to the discussion in his own voice.)

For the presenters onstage and for the audience, it is an interesting dance, especially if one does not know Tibetan. It is helpful to simply rest in the present moment, rather than busying oneself with thoughts. It is a meditation in its own right to stay present and not become impatient or distracted at those times, because in the very next moment, the conversation is likely to be taken up once again or turn to an important point that needs clarification from the presenter so that His Holiness and others can understand what is being suggested or demonstrated.

Immediately to the Dalai Lama's right is the chair that each presenter occupies for his or her presentation. That way, the presenter is right next to the Dalai Lama and is able to speak directly to him in a way that resembles an intimate conversation rather than a formal lecture. Frequent eye contact and laughter between His Holiness and the presenter often punctuate these conversations. It is a very intimate setting in which both goodwill and deep engagement in the question at hand tend to spread rapidly to include all the other participants in that session, as well as the observers in the room.

It was that intimacy and warmth that we hoped to capture on the stage of Constitution Hall by keeping more or less the same format, in a sense replicating His Holiness's living room in front of three thousand people. Some of the photographs included in this volume convey the cozy atmosphere of this setting. Large video screens on either side of the stage ensured that the speakers would be visible from the back of the hall, in hopes that even in such a large group each individual would feel a vital part of the conversation, a true colleague and participant in his or her own right.

To that end, on a number of occasions Richie and Jon, as cohosts, invited audience members to reflect on how essential they were to this meeting, in ways both known and unknown at that moment in time. Their presence, their deep listening, their questions, and, most of all, their motivation and unique reasons for being there might encourage them to probe more deeply into their own hunches or assumptions, and perhaps open up new possibilities for research or clinical applications in their areas of interest and expertise. The audience had been selected through a web-based application process that favored clinicians, researchers, scholars, and students in the biological and neurosciences, including medical and graduate students—an ideal audience to make the maximal impact on a nascent and rapidly growing field.

THE MEETING GETS UNDER WAY

Adam Engle, cofounder with Francisco Varela of the Mind and Life Institute, and its president and CEO, opens the meeting with welcoming remarks.

Adam Engle: Your Holiness, Father Thomas, President DeGioia, Dean Miller, distinguished scientists, clinicians, and brothers and sisters, eighteen years ago the Dalai Lama, Francisco Varela, and I embarked upon an experiment to see if we could create a methodology whereby scientists, philosophers, and Buddhist contemplatives could come together in a joint quest for a more complete understanding of the nature of reality, for investigating the mind, and for promoting well-being on the planet. Since 1987, the Mind and Life Dialogues have covered many topics upon which scientists and contemplatives have shared their findings and enriched each other's understanding, ranging from physics and cosmology to neuroplasticity, and from healing emotions to altruism and ethics.

Today we take another step forward on this journey. On behalf of the Dalai Lama and the other members of the board of the Mind and Life Institute, I welcome you all to Mind and Life XIII, "The Science and Clinical Applications of Meditation."

The topic for this meeting comes from the recognition that our work at the Mind and Life Institute is no longer limited to dialogue and understanding. More important is the need to translate these understandings into programs, interventions, and tools that will bring tangible benefit into peoples' lives. Hence, we have begun to ask very practical questions: How do we nurture and maintain healthy minds? How can we cultivate more emotional balance in our lives and in our societies? And how can we teach these self-management skills earlier in life?

Currently the Mind and Life Institute operates through four divisions, all working together to promote scientific understanding and individual and cultural well-being. Our Mind and Life Dialogues with the Dalai Lama set the scientific agenda by exploring which areas of science are most ripe for collaboration with contemplatives and how that collaboration can be implemented most effectively. Our Mind and Life publications report to the greater scientific community and the interested public on what has occurred in our dialogues. Our Mind and Life Summer Research Institute is an annual, weeklong residential symposium retreat for researchers and practitioners of science, contemplation, and philosophy to explore how to advance the hypotheses formulated at the Mind and Life Dialogues and the Institute's research initiatives. Our Mind and Life research grant program provides seed research grants to investigate the hypotheses thus formulated and explored.

In the short time we have together over the next two and a half days, we will only begin to explore how we can more skillfully use the techniques of meditation and other forms of mental training in clinical applications to improve health and well-being. It is our deepest desire that you—both the audience and the participants—become inspired to explore and expand this frontier in your own lives and work.

I thank the Georgetown University Medical Center and the Johns Hopkins University School of Medicine for joining us in sponsoring this dialogue and for their leadership in integrative medical research. I thank the speakers and panelists for their wisdom, kindness, and insight, and the many days of preparation they have devoted to make this symposium beneficial. I thank our sustaining patrons and our gold and silver sponsors, who provided financial support to make this meeting possible. Most importantly, I thank each and every one of you for your interest and openness in joining this exploration.

Adam then invites both Edward Miller, MD, dean of the Johns Hopkins University School of Medicine, and John DeGioia, president of Georgetown University, to make opening remarks. Each cites his institution's commitment to the new field of integrative medicine and speak to the role that scientific evidence plays in providing a foundation for the development of new treatment approaches to patient care, including the increasingly prevalent meditation-based approaches. President DeGioia then introduces His Holiness.

John DeGioia: It is my great privilege this morning to introduce the Mind and Life Institute's honorary chairman and continuing inspiration, His Holiness the Dalai Lama. One can hardly imagine a more extraordinary life than that of the gentleman we are about to meet. He was born on a modest farm in the mountains of Tibet. In this remote nation a distinctive form of Buddhism has developed, along with the belief that the Buddha is reincarnated as the Dalai Lama in order to lead others to enlightenment, and to serve as the spiritual and temporal leader of Tibet.

After the death of the thirteenth Dalai Lama in 1933, a group of holy men began a secret search for the next Dalai Lama. In time that search brought them to a peasant family with a precocious two-year-old boy. Based on a variety of tests, the holy men determined that this youngster was the fourteenth Dalai Lama. Like his predecessors for centuries before him, the child and his family were taken to the capital city, where crowds cheered his arrival. At the age of six he was enthroned as the spiritual leader of his people and took the name Tenzin Gyatso. He lived in the Potala Palace, its thousand rooms a source of endless fascination for a curious boy.

At age sixteen, two years ahead of schedule, the Dalai Lama assumed full control of Tibet after his nation was invaded by the Chinese army. For nine years he worked to negotiate a peaceful resolution, but in 1959 a deteriorating situation convinced His Holiness to seek political asylum in India. From there he leads the Tibetan government in exile and more than 120,000 Tibetans who are living as exiles. He established schools and heritage centers to keep Tibetan culture alive and reformed the government in exile along democratic lines.

For decades the Dalai Lama has traveled the world to seek support for his proposals to bring a nonviolent solution to the situation in Tibet. He's been an eloquent voice for human rights and world peace, and the world's foremost exponent of Buddhist philosophy. In 1989, he received the Nobel Peace Prize for his advocacy on behalf of his homeland.

It is an extraordinary life, to be sure, but today we see another aspect of this remarkable man. The Dalai Lama's early education was extensive in many areas, but he was not exposed to math, physics, biology, or other sciences. Yet he was an inquisitive child who was fascinated by several mechanical objects that he found in the palace. In time and with travel, his interests broadened to include all aspects of science and the scientific form of inquiry. He has taken the opportunity to get to know some of the most distinguished scientists of our time, to discuss progress in scientific thinking, and to explore the interface between faith and science. He shares many of his insights in his new book, *The Universe in a Single Atom: The Convergence of Science and Spirituality.*[13]

Today the Dalai Lama stands at the forefront of the dialogue between science and spirituality. The conversation, he believes, has enormous potential to help the human family meet unprecedented global challenges. Please join me this morning in welcoming His Holiness the Dalai Lama.

Thus begins the three days of presentations and dialogue. We hope that the meeting will come alive for you, the reader, as you explore these presentations. We hope that in one way or another, because of the give-and-take and the somewhat informal nature of the talks and conversations, you will be transported into the room and feel the energy of the presentations as they unfold and engender dialogue among the presenters, panelists, and His Holiness.

Before His Holiness rose to make his opening remarks from the podium, Adam Engle put up a photograph of our dear friend and colleague Francisco Varela (1946–2001). Francisco had been the guiding scientific light and inspiration of the Mind and Life Institute from its very beginning, and had grown extremely close to His Holiness over the years. His untimely death at the age of fifty-five was a huge loss for the Mind and Life community. That loss was felt and shared by all who knew this remarkable polymath of a human being, with his incredible intellect and equally incredible heart. Francisco was a deep and devoted Buddhist practitioner and a student of some of the greatest Tibetan lamas of the day. We were uplifted, however, by the continuing unfolding and evolution of his vision and legacy at the Mind and Life Institute, as well by as the enduring imprint of his research and writings on the world. We dedicated the meeting to his memory.

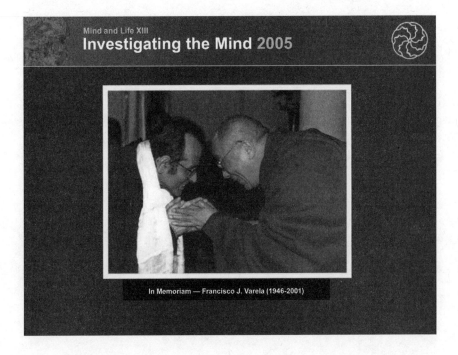

Mind and Life XIII
Investigating the Mind 2005

In Memoriam — Francisco J. Varela (1946-2001)

SESSION 1

MEDITATION-BASED CLINICAL INTERVENTIONS: SCIENCE, PRACTICE, AND IMPLEMENTATION

The first session sets the stage for the rest of the meeting. His Holiness opens the session with cogent introductory remarks that highlight his interest in and respect for science and his interest in brain research. Richard Davidson and Jon Kabat-Zinn then offer welcoming remarks. The first presentation outlines the Buddhist perspective on suffering, liberation from suffering, and universal qualities of the human mind. The second and third presentations discuss clinical and research programs exploring the impacts of meditation on patients with chronic health conditions and on neural activity and various physiological functions. The moderator for this session is Matthieu Ricard.

HH Dalai Lama: I am very happy to have this opportunity to participate in the thirteenth Mind and Life Dialogue, and I would like to express my deep appreciation to all the participants and the panelists. I am already familiar with some of the scientists who are going to participate in this dialogue, and there are also going to be a few new scientists and, of course, the contemplative practitioners as well. So I'd like to take the opportunity to express my appreciation to all of you first.

One thing that is unique to this particular Mind and Life Dialogue is the presence of Father Thomas Keating, who represents the Christian spiritual tradition. It's a particularly great source of joy for me to have that important spiritual tradition represented, and I would like to welcome you to this dialogue. In fact, I have expressed a wish on several occasions during these Mind and Life conferences that, since contemplative practice is not unique to the Buddhist tradition but rather a common spiritual practice that spans a wide range of the world's spiritual traditions, it would be beneficial if some of these other spiritual traditions could also be represented in these dialogues.

When I saw the picture of Francisco Varela, who is no longer with us—as soon as I heard Adam mention his name I pictured his face, particularly his large, shining forehead and his eyes, which were always very alert. Although he is no longer with us, his work and his vision are still very much alive. I think that's important. Sometimes certain noble work depends entirely on one individual. So long as that individual is there, that work is active. Once that individual is no longer there, then his or her work also eventually diminishes. I think that's unfortunate. So I'm very happy now that certain work initiated by our friend not only still continues, but seems to be growing. I really appreciate all of the people who make every effort to continue that noble work.

One of the unique things about Buddhism, particularly in the Sanskrit tradition, is that investigation and experiment play a very important part. Many troubles come out of ignorance, and the only antidote to ignorance is knowledge. Knowledge means a clear understanding of reality, which must come through investigation and experiment. In ancient times, the Nalanda masters[14] carried out these investigations mainly through logic and human thought, and perhaps in some cases through meditation. In modern times, there is another way to find out about reality: with help of equipment. I think both science and Buddhist investigation are actually trying to find reality.

Furthermore, there is a tradition in Buddhism that if we find something that contradicts our scripture, we have the liberty to reject that scripture. That gives us a kind of freedom to investigate, regardless of what the literature says. For example, there are some descriptions of cosmology in the scriptures that are quite a disgrace. When I give teachings to Buddhist audiences, I often tell them that we cannot accept these things.

In the initial stages of my curiosity, I would look out into space and see many things. I was curious how these things came to be. Look at our body. There's a lot of hair on the head and, underneath it, a skull. Unlike other parts of the body, there is some kind of special protection there. Why? Usually we believe the soul or self lies at the center of the heart. Now it seems that the soul—if we can identify it at all—is here in the head, not in the heart.

The Buddhist texts on psychology and epistemology make a clear distinction between two qualitatively different domains of experience. One is the sensory level: our experience of the five senses. The other is what Buddhists refer to as the mental level of experience: thoughts, emotions, and so on. The primary seat, or physical basis, of sensory experience is thought to be the sensory organs themselves. But now it seems to be clear from modern neuroscience that the central organizing principle of sensory experience is really to be found more in the brain than in the sensory organs themselves.

Buddhists are very interested to learn such things from scientific findings. I think the relationship is very helpful. Therefore, we began introducing the study of science to selected Buddhist monastic students in India more than four years ago. A systematic introduction of science education in the monastic curriculum is gradually being established.

As for my participation here, I have nothing to offer. I am always eager just to listen and learn from these great, experienced scientists. Although there is a language problem, and also my memory problem, it sometimes seems that I learn from the session—but after the session there is nothing left in my head. So there's the problem! Anyway, it may leave some imprints in my brain.

Richard Davidson: Jon Kabat-Zinn and I are the scientific coordinators of this meeting, and it's a pleasure for us to welcome you. I'd like to take this opportunity to underscore my excitement about this dialogue and about the potential of the interaction between scientists and contemplatives. One of the themes that you'll be hearing repeatedly over the next two and half days is the idea that there are certain positive qualities, such as happiness and compassion, that the contemplative traditions teach us are not fixed characteristics. We are not indelibly fixed in our current state, but rather these are characteristics that can be transformed. There is a very precious and important convergence of that idea with the modern concept of neuroplasticity—the notion that the brain can change in response to experience and training—a convergence that provides a foundation for us as scientists to go forward in a truly novel and integrative way.

We'll also be hearing about the idea that transforming the mind and the brain may transform certain aspects of the body, which can have potentially positive effects on at least some aspects of our health.

So we're in for a very exciting two and a half days—and more than just exciting. I think this is a historic occasion. It is our hope and conviction that this meeting will propel a new kind of science forward.

Jon Kabat-Zinn: At His Holiness's express request, our intent with this meeting is to have a much larger conversation than we have been able to hold in the past, one that might touch many more people than even the books that have been published about the private meetings could reach. People who care deeply about these issues from the point of view of basic science, of clinical applications, of applications to one's own life, all of which are coextensive, have gathered here today to participate in deep and meaningful ways. Ripples will go out from this gathering. The invitation is meant to be truly participatory; this is a collective investigation in which you, the audience, play an extremely important role.

One way that you can participate is through deep listening and letting the veil of expectations drop away for a time. It's very easy to be disappointed if your particular area of interest doesn't get touched on to the degree you would like, but there's something else happening that's much larger than that, part of which has to do with non-attachment. We're all, in some sense, engaged in a meditative process simply by being here. You will also be able to participate by asking questions of the presenters and panelists, and we'll do our best to respond to them collectively. Of course, His Holiness will be the first responder of choice, in every sense of that term.

I offer another deep bow of welcome to you. I think there is an element of mystery in who shows up in a room like this. You have come from all over the world to be here. We don't know what the outcome of this gathering will be, but in a sense, what is happening is that a community of practice—what Buddhists call a sangha—is expressing itself, and its members are getting a chance to look at and experience each other. Much of what is most important in these conferences happens among you in the interim times, in the conversations and new friendships that develop, and in the deep inquiry into the nature of the subject matter at hand. So, welcome one and welcome all.

Matthieu Ricard: This morning we are going to reflect on the nature of meditation, the principle of applying mindfulness-based meditation to better well-being, and how meditation can be studied in collaboration with neuroscience.

One of the first questions we ask ourselves is why bother to meditate, and if we do, on what, and how? The very nature of meditation is mental training, a tool of transformation over the long term of our life. We should understand that mental health is not simply the absence of mental illness. Are we really living our life in the most optimal way? Is what we call our "normal" state of going about life really optimal? We can see from our own experience that the way we engage with and interpret the world is often distorted by a mode of perception that doesn't correspond with the way things are. Often we find ourselves in the pangs of torment from mental toxins such as hatred, obsessive desire, arrogance, nagging jealousy. Those are certainly not optimal ways of relating to our own experience or to others. We know that we can experience genuine altruistic love and compassion, but couldn't we do so more often, so that those states of mind become the normal way we relate to others? Hence the ideal of long-term transformation: becoming a better human being for one's own well-being and that of others as well. These two go together.

That is precisely the meaning of meditation. Meditation is not just sitting and blissing out under a mango tree in order to have a better day, although it might help. If we look at the Eastern roots of the word for meditation, it truly means cultivation—cultivating new qualities, new ways of being. It also means familiarization: familiarization with a new way of seeing the world; for example, not grasping at permanence, and instead seeing the dynamic flow of interdependence. Meditation means familiarization with qualities that we have the potential to enhance, like unconditional compassion, openness to others, and inner peace. It's also familiarization with the very way the mind works. So often we are full of thoughts that ceaselessly go through our mind. We hardly notice what's going on. What is behind the screen of thoughts? Can we relate to some kind of basic mindfulness and open presence?

All of these sorts of inner exploration are considered meditation. From the start, the Buddhist path has a therapeutic goal: to free ourselves and others from suffering. Obviously this is not a mere hobby, something nice to add to our lives. Rather, inner transformation is something that determines the quality of every instant we live.

Still, we may ask why there is a need for the contemplative traditions to collaborate with science. What can both sides expect? What can humanity expect from that?

For those who have been engaged in this process of mental transformation, the benefits are obvious (hopefully, if our practice goes well). This creates a wish to share something dear to ourselves, which has brought so much to our lives and could do the same for others.

Collaborating with science also speaks to the aspiration to know things as they are. We know about the experience of specific states of meditation, but what is their signature in the brain? What is the relation of different states of meditation with other known cognitive and emotional states that have been studied in the mind and the brain? What might the effects of long-term mind training be? We know that learning to play a musical instrument, for instance, can change your brain. It's wonderful to play the piano, though it's not a major deficit if you don't. But compassion, attention, vigilance, mindfulness, inner peace—these are fundamental aspects of the quality of our life, and it is quite sad if we don't develop them to their optimal point.

The hope of this dialogue is to increase and deepen our knowledge of both what mental training really is and how it affects the brain, the body, and our relation to the world and to others in the short term and the long term. How will that eventually be a contribution to humanity? That is truly our common goal. Can we contribute something to education through cultivating emotional balance? As His Holiness often says, we cannot have outer peace without inner peace. We cannot have an outer disarmament without inner disarmament. If we want to have a harmonious society, it has to begin with and within each of us. That is what meditation is about, and that's what we are going to hear about this morning. First, Ajahn Amaro will delineate some of the main principles of meditation, mind training, and the Buddhist path.

AJAHN AMARO *How Buddhist Meditative Practices Can Inform Our Understanding of Pain and Suffering, the Potential for Healing, the Relief of Suffering, and the Underlying Nature of the Human Mind and Body*

> *Distinctions between pain and suffering are critical and relevant within the context of Buddhist thought and practice. This talk maps out a Buddhist perspective on suffering, its ultimate causes, the possibility of liberation from suffering, and a systematic path for doing so. It also touches on what Buddhists refer to as universal qualities of the human mind—qualities that are directly accessible through the cultivation of awareness by means of meditation.*

I have been invited to give an outline of some of the principle themes of Buddhist teachings, particularly concerning the nature of the common, almost universal, human experience of suffering—what we call dukkha, or dissatisfaction—and its relation to meditation.

Before beginning I should underscore the fact that Buddhist teachings and ideas are traditionally always presented in the spirit of being offered for consideration and reflection rather than being held up as dogma that the listener is expected to believe. They are themes that one is invited to listen to; to take in, as His Holiness was encouraging; to contemplate; and to reflect on. That which is useful, one is encouraged to take and retain; that which we feel is wrong or doesn't match our experience, we can leave aside; and that of which we are uncertain can be left on the "maybe" shelf.

Just as doctors, pharmacologists, and medical researchers exist because we don't experience perfect health all the time, similarly it could be said that psychotherapies, spiritual teachings, and religions exist because we don't experience perfect happiness all the time, even when social or physical conditions are ideal, to say nothing of when we are challenged. For example, I just flew in from England a couple of days ago, so I woke up bright and breezy at 2:15 this morning. There I was in the Hyatt Grand Hotel, with those sparkling fountains and the beautiful, rich foliage of the houseplants and the glorious, palatial space, but my mind was capable of getting into a state, thinking, "Oh dear, it's 2:15 in the morning. I haven't

27

had enough rest! I've got to give a presentation today!" Yet there I was, in extreme comfort. In the cabin where I live in the forest at my monastery, I don't even have electricity or an indoor toilet. So there I was in ideal conditions, yet my mind could get caught up, worried, anxious, distressed. This is what we mean by the quality of dukkha, or dissatisfaction: the capacity of the mind to lose its balance, to become emotionally stressed.

The Buddha's teaching is somewhat unusual among world religions insofar as it is not centered around any kind of metaphysical statements. Essentially, the Buddha was a pragmatist, and so he aimed his attention primarily at this experience of dissatisfaction and suffering, or dukkha in the scriptural language. This was his focus. Even though he was a theoretician as well, with immense capacity to understand how the world worked, he limited his teaching to what would be practical for people. This is much more a clinician's approach to knowledge about the body and the mind than a researcher's. The Buddha focused on the precise things that help us on a practical, day-to-day basis, rather than the entire field of knowledge.

There's a famous analogy he gave one time: He reached down to the floor of the forest where he was walking with some of his monks, picked up a handful of leaves, and said, "Which is the greater in number, the leaves in my hand or the leaves in the forest?" The monks with him said, "Of course the number of leaves in your hand is very small, and the number of leaves in the forest is very, very great." The Buddha said, "Similarly, what I know could be compared to the leaves in the forest. What I teach you is comparable to what I hold in my hand. And why do I only teach you this limited range? Because these are the things that will help to bring you happiness, to bring you true peace, to bring you liberation from dissatisfaction." The other stuff may be true, but it is not immediately helpful for healing spiritual or psychological ailments.

The Buddha used another analogy, a simile of the wounded soldier: A soldier is shot with a poisoned arrow on the battlefield. The field surgeon comes and is about to pull the arrow out, but the soldier says, "Oh no, don't pull the arrow out until you find out the name of the person who shot me. I also need to know the name of the village that he came from. Not only that, I need to know the names of his parents and his grandparents on both sides. I need to know the kind of wood the arrow was made from. I need to know the kind of tip the arrow was fitted with and how it was bound onto the shaft of the arrow. I need to know the kind of bird the feather came from. Is it a goose feather? Is it a peacock feather? Is it a chicken feather? Is it a duck feather?" The Buddha goes on this long extrapolation until we get the point: By the time the surgeon has answered all the questions, the soldier will surely be dead. The point, he said, is to pull out the arrow and dress the wound. That's what the emphasis is in the Buddhist tradition, to try to address the central element of dissatisfaction, this quality of dukkha.

One of the epithets the Buddha acquired over the years was "the Doctor of the World." A reason for this is that the central insight and framework that he taught, known as the Four Noble Truths, is cast in the formulation of a classical Indian medical diagnosis. The format begins with the nature of the symptom. In this particular kind of psychological or spiritual disease, the symptom is dukkha, the experience of dissatisfaction; this is the First Noble Truth. The second element in this diagnostic format is the cause of that symptom, which the Buddha outlined as being self-centered craving, greed, hatred, and delusion. These are the toxins that Matthieu referred to, the negative afflictive emotions, habits, and qualities that the mind gets caught up in and that poison the heart; this is the Second Noble Truth. The third element is the prognosis, and the good news is that it is curable. This is the Third Noble Truth, that the experience of dissatisfaction can end; we can be free from it. The fourth element—and the Fourth Noble Truth—is the methodology of treatment: what the Buddha laid out as the way to heal this wound. It's known in some expressions as the Eightfold Path, but it can be outlined in three fundamental elements: first, responsible behavior or virtue, living a moral and ethical life; second, mental collectedness, meditation, and mind training; and third, the development of insightful understanding in accordance with reality, or wisdom. These three elements are the fundamental treatment for this psychological, spiritual ailment of dissatisfaction.

I should underline that the Buddha didn't make any claim to have a monopoly on truth. When somebody once asked him, "Is it the case that you're the only one who really understands the way things are, and that all other spiritual teachings are incorrect, all other paths are erroneous?" He said, "No, by no means." It's not a matter of the way the teachings are framed, the language or symbolism that one uses. It is simply the presence or absence of these three central qualities: ethical behavior, mental collectedness, and wisdom. If any spiritual path contains those three elements, then it will certainly lead to the possibility and the actuality of freedom, peace, a harmony within oneself, and an easefulness in life. If it doesn't contain those elements, then it cannot lead to easefulness, peace, and liberation.

I'm very glad that Father Thomas is here representing the Christian contemplative tradition. This is in keeping with His Holiness's ecumenical spirit, respecting very deeply that the Buddhist tradition makes no claim to exclusive knowledge of the true way, but instead celebrates whatever pathways we find, whether we call them religions or psychotherapies or something else, that help bring to our lives a quality of happiness, to enable ourselves and others to live more peacefully and fully.

In using the word "dissatisfaction" or "dukkha," a theme that will probably inform the discussion throughout this gathering is that there are two dimensions to this experience. The Buddha outlines these very clearly. The first is that the experience of physical and emotional pain is inescapable, endemic in our very lives as human beings and intrinsic to the fact that we have a body and a mind. We can call this natural suffering or, more simply, pain. The main focus of the Buddha's teaching was on a second element, which we call adventitious suffering: what the mind adds to a negative experience. When we feel physical pain or have some kind of difficulty, the fretfulness, resistance, resentment, and anxiety we create around the experience is this second kind of suffering.

The Buddha used another analogy about being shot by an arrow. (By the way, the Buddha was a warrior noble, so there's a lot of military language in his teaching.) The Buddha said that when you experience physical pain, it's like being shot by an arrow. When, on top of that physical pain, you resist it and resent it, it's like being shot by a second arrow.

If we're unwise, then most often the only way we know how to deal with pain is to escape from it through absorbing the mind into something pleasurable, which leads to the blind pursuit of sensory pleasure. Yet that contributes to a greater sense of stress and dislocation.

Another important point is that we can make problems not just in response to negative or painful experiences. Adventitious suffering occurs not just in response to physical or emotional pain. We certainly do experience many kinds of natural emotional pain; for example, losing someone we love or, within this company, submitting an academic paper for publication and being rejected by our journal of choice. Grief can arise from such experiences. But we are capable of creating suffering even out of plea-surable experiences. We can have something that's extremely beautiful and desirable, something we absolutely wanted and chose—like getting that paper published in that wonderful journal. But then five, ten, or twenty years go by and depression sets in: "Well, I was really great back in the eighties, but what have I done since then?" The thing that was rejoiced in, being a star, becomes a knife twisting in the wound twenty years later. Even pleasurable experiences contain within them the seed of dissatisfac-tion if we relate to them unwisely.

Pain, the first kind of suffering or dissatisfaction, is endemic and unavoidable. The second kind is completely eradicable, as the Buddha suggested in his teachings and from his own experience. This is something that we as individuals can discover for ourselves. This is the good news of the Third Noble Truth: adventitious suffering can end. Even when we have a painful experience, whether physical or emotional, a headache or some great loss, the heart and mind can still be completely at peace with it. It can be seen as absolutely okay, with no struggle against it, no resis-tance or resentment. There is no suffering or dissatisfaction created around it. This is a key element of Buddhist spiritual and psychological training. It will be described in many presentations during this meeting.

To expand a little on what Matthieu was saying, meditation would be defined as the refinement of innate abilities that we already possess. Sometimes the word "meditation" can be loaded with all kinds of precon-ceptions that we've picked up from different TV shows, popular magazines, news, or gossip. But from the classical Buddhist perspective, meditation isn't an attempt to have any particularly special experience or strange vision or acquire special abilities. It's more like working with a couple of innate capacities that the mind possesses: the ability to focus the attention and the capacity to investigate, explore, and contemplate the nature of experience itself. These two capacities are natural to us, and meditation develops them, like cultivating a seed and giving it the conditions to grow and flourish. That is the purpose and the nature of meditation.

To give an example, in one of the most common forms of meditation, we take a simple, natural object such as the rhythm of our own breath as it unfolds moment by moment, which is calming and relatively easily felt. By sitting down, closing the eyes, and focusing the attention on one's breathing, over time and with effort and application, the breath becomes what we call a meditation object. The mind is trained to attend to that simple, unexciting stimulus. That quality of attention can be developed so that the mind rests more and more easily in the present moment and stays with that object. The more the attention is trained on the present, the more we are able to break the habit of being dragged around by compulsions and distractions—the mind constantly creating scenarios for the future, rewriting the past, being lost in distracted thought, or subjected to incessant reams of thinking. Most of us here have had those times where it seems like nothing can make the mind stop. It just goes on and on and on and on and on. The capacity to focus in meditation has a lot to do with learning how to think when we choose to think, and learning how not to think when we choose not to.

The second capacity, the element of investigation, supports a quality of understanding. We learn to see how the mind works: its habits of reaction, running away from the painful, chasing after the pleasurable, and becoming bored, irritated, or restless with the neutral. By recognizing those habits and knowing them fully through the capacity of focus, we learn how not to be drawn into the compulsive cycles that come with them.

An analogy that comes to mind is using a camera. Picking up the camera and holding it is like the qualities of responsible behavior and virtue: wisely picking up and holding your life. Focusing the lens is like the development of concentration. Framing the precise shot that you want to make is the element of wisdom. Actually snapping the picture brings the delight that comes with having caught a fine image—that pleasing quality of catching the moment in that way: "Yes! Got it!" This is similar to the insight and transformation that occur when we see the world in a different, more emotionally balanced way.

I'd like to address a common misunderstanding about meditation. We often think about relaxation as being zoned out, a sort of lazy-boy mode, where you slide back, thinking, "I'm going to relax." It's almost synonymous with dozing off or going into a semiconscious state. We also like the stimulation of being aroused, interested, or excited—the excitement of a roller coaster or scary movie. Some of the other presentations will address research into the short-term stress associated with that quality of stimulation we love.

One of the characteristics of Buddhist meditation that we can discover for ourselves is that, perhaps surprisingly, relaxation and arousal are not mutually exclusive. When the mind is truly alert, fully attentive to the present moment with a clear, unwavering focus, whether one is attending to the breath or not, it can be completely peaceful and highly energetic at the same time. The two are not mutually exclusive. You may think, "Wait a minute. That's not the way I've experienced things." That's fine; for each of us, our personal experience is the final arbiter of truth. But I offer the suggestion that you suspend disbelief if you can. Maybe it is possible. Take a look for yourself and see.

In the Buddhist tradition, the quality of ease of being and the understanding of the nature of our life—what we call in our vernacular liberation or enlightenment—is the standard for perfect mental health. In the Buddhist tradition, you're not completely sane until you're fully enlightened. The familiar conditions of compulsively running away from the painful, pursuing the pleasant, and getting bored with the neutral—the coping strategies you might consider to be normal conduct or indicative of sanity—are considered in Buddhist psychology a less than fully sane state of mind. It's interesting to compare the models of Buddhist and Western psychology in this respect.

The last point I'd like to address is the relationship between our physical and psychological aspects, particularly in how the mind relates to physical pain and the effect that pain can have on both mind and body. Take the example of sitting meditation. In an ordinary period of meditation practice in the monastery where I live, we sit for forty-five minutes. When you sit with your body in a cross-legged posture, completely still for three-quarters of an hour, it's very easy to experience aching knees or pain in various parts of the body. As that painful sensation starts to arise in the body, the initial reactive pattern can be "I'm trying to concentrate on my breath. This pain in my knee is getting in the way. I wish it would go away. Oh dear, is that my meniscus ripping? I'm going to need knee surgery. Oh my god, they're going to have to carry me out of here on a stretcher." The body tenses up and feelings of aversion, fear, and anxiety cluster around that painful feeling like a swarm of flies around a piece of meat.

If you recognize what is happening—that a negative reactive process of adventitious suffering is clustering around that sensation—you will find that you can work with it in at least two different modes, applying the principles I've been describing. First, you could relax the attitude, recognizing, for example, that this is just a feeling of pain in your knee and you probably won't need surgery today. It's just a discomfort that arose only a couple of minutes ago, so perhaps it's not absolutely life threatening at the moment. You can probably live with it for the next five minutes without any kind of danger. No need to get upset. No need to get anxious. Relax, let go, and soften the attitude.

The second part is relaxing the body, noticing that, while you've been reacting blindly to the painful sensation, the knee, the hip joints, and the back have all tensed up. Physically relaxing the body and your attitude toward the experience of strong unpleasant sensation has two effects. The first is that the subjective degree of pain actually diminishes. If it was a pain level of six out of ten, relaxing the body causes it to drop to a, say, three out of ten. Then, even though it's still a level-three pain, by relaxing your attitude toward it—and this is the key point—you can recognize it as not being a problem. There's a complete peacefulness and ease even though the pain is present.

I'm just putting this out as a suggestion. It is certainly a common experience in Buddhist meditation, and I've experienced it myself. A crucial element is recognizing that one can experience pain on a physical basis and still be completely at peace with it. The most useful element is when we transfer that recognition to emotional pain, as well.

For instance, you can experience the grief of your paper not being published or, as a doctor, of having a patient die that you treated in the best way you could, or whatever it might be. There can be a complete ease with even that degree of emotional pain. There is a way of being with uncomfortable experiences, knowing them, and letting them be, so that we find ourselves more able to live in harmony with all of those different dimensions of life.

Matthieu Ricard: Thank you, Ajahn Amaro, for that orientation to some of the basic framework we will be discussing throughout this dialogue. Building on that foundation, we will now take a look at how meditation and its fundamental aspect of mindfulness can help or affect our daily life. For many years, Jon Kabat-Zinn has been trying to see how bringing more mindfulness into our way of being can help people who are suffering, whether physically or mentally. His presentation will explain some of his work in regard to mindfulness-based meditation.

JON KABAT-ZINN *Some Clinical Applications of Mindfulness Meditation in Medicine and Psychiatry: The Case of Mindfulness-Based Stress Reduction (MBSR)*

Since 1979, mindfulness-based stress reduction (MBSR) has become widely accepted, used, and studied within mainstream medicine and psychiatry. This presentation describes MBSR's approach to making mindfulness, the foundational core of Buddhist meditation, accessible to Western medical patients in a secular form while preserving the universal dharma dimension at its heart. Results from two clinical trials are presented, one on rates of skin clearing in psoriasis, the other on emotional processing in cortical regions of the brain and accompanying effects on immune function. Directions in current and future research programs are considered.

Your Holiness, I would like to speak with you this morning about work that my colleagues and I have been doing at the University of Massachusetts Medical School for many years now. Some of my colleagues are in the audience this morning, as are many others who have also been doing this kind of work elsewhere.

At the heart of MBSR is an experiment to see whether we could take the essence of Buddhist meditation practice, insofar as we understand it, and somehow make it accessible to people who would not find it through a traditional Buddhist or spiritual path, but who nevertheless are plagued by suffering and dukkha. As you yourself so often point out, suffering is a universal phenomenon. Our minds are all basically the same. Our bodies are all basically the same. If there was some way to translate the Buddhadharma so that it did not lose its essential dimensions, but became available to be heard and enacted or embodied by regular people who are not particularly interested in either Buddhism or meditation, it might potentially be beneficial. That was the challenge, if you will, the experiment.

Somebody asked Your Holiness during the press conference, "I know a lot of people meditate, but I can't. Do you find that many people can't meditate?" We have tried to design the MBSR program specifically for people who think they can't meditate. That's just another idea or opinion. Often people have very strange ideas about what meditation is.

I will describe what we call mindfulness-based stress reduction, the rationale and motivation behind it, how we understand and use the term "mindfulness," how this approach has spread, and its integration into medicine nowadays. I will very briefly describe one outcome study on the effect of the mind on the body. And although I will not cover this in my talk, I want to invite discussion on what characteristics and standards are needed to do this translational work in a way that has integrity.

Ajahn Amaro spoke of the framing of the Four Noble Truths in what is basically a medical format: a diagnosis of dukkha, a cause or an etiology, a prognosis, and a treatment. I have found many links between medicine and meditation. In English, the two words sound very much alike, and in fact, as your old friend David Bohm pointed out in his wonderful book *Wholeness and the Implicate Order*,[15] the words "meditation" and "medicine" come from the same Indo-European root, which means "to measure," in the Platonic sense of everything having its own right inward measure. Medicine is the restoring of right inward measure or balance when it's disrupted, and meditation is the direct perceiving of right, inward measure in all phenomena.

Just as there are vows in Buddhism, such as the bodhisattva vow to save all sentient beings, in medicine doctors also take a formal vow, called the Hippocratic Oath: a vow to put one's personal concerns and interests last and the patient's concerns and interests first. The cardinal principle of the Hippocratic Oath is "First do no harm." Non-harming is a profound ethical stance that requires some degree of selflessness. So medicine and meditation, in their traditional guises, actually have a great deal in common.

Hospitals obviously are refuges for people who are suffering. Because of this, we sometimes refer to them as "dukkha magnets." What better place to develop and offer a universal dharma approach for the relief of suffering and to investigate its clinical effectiveness?

We call what we do stress reduction because everybody can relate to that: "Stress—I get that; I can understand it. I need my stress reduced." Interestingly, some Buddhist scholars who translate Pali into English are now using the term "stress" rather than "suffering" as a translation of dukkha.

Stress can be either acute or chronic. Medicine handles acute stress very well, whether in the hospital emergency room or in psychiatric emergencies. That is not what the Stress Reduction Clinic is for. The Stress Reduction Clinic is for people who have long-term chronic difficulties that medicine has not been able to alleviate completely. In fact, many people fall through the cracks of the health care system to one degree or another and do not receive total satisfaction in terms of their medical conditions and health concerns, which just compounds the dukkha they experience. The Stress Reduction Clinic can serve as a refuge for people with chronic medical conditions and chronic stress at critical times in their lives.

When people feel very stressed, they often say, "This experience is taking years off my life." Now there is scientific proof that this actually is the case. Certain kinds of suffering have been shown to increase the rate at which telomeres are shortened. Telomeres are the repeat DNA subunits at the ends of our chromosomes. They are involved in cell division, and how rapidly they are degraded appears to be tied to the rate at which we age biologically. So stress reduction becomes a potentially important vehicle for helping people reestablish balance and well-being in their lives, as a complement to whatever the doctors are able to do for them.

Since we call what we do mindfulness-based stress reduction, it's fair to ask what mindfulness is. I don't need to say much about it after Ajahn Amaro's elegant presentation. As you well know, mindfulness is often spoken of as the heart of Buddhist meditation. And as Your Holiness has often pointed out, in all East Asian languages, including Tibetan, the word for mind is the same as the word for heart. In the MBSR programs, we try to emphasize that the word "mindfulness" equally means "heartfulness." Our operational definition of mindfulness is "moment-to-moment non-judgmental awareness, cultivated by purposely paying attention in the present moment." Kindness and self-compassion are an intimate part of the attending.

I will briefly sketch out the MBSR program. I don't need to go into it in great detail, because it has been described extensively. What we're trying to do is create an environment where people can learn to slow down in their lives—or maybe even stop—and familiarize themselves with stilling the body, observing what is going on in both body and mind, and cultivating a certain kind of intimacy with the present moment as it is. Most of the time people are surprised to discover, when they start to pay attention in this way, that they have not been living in the present moment. We live mostly in the future, worrying or planning, or in the past, remembering things that happened before, and sometimes getting quite bent out of shape about them. In Western societies, stopping can be a radical act in and of itself. I believe that just stopping and opening one's field of awareness is, ultimately, a radical act of self-compassion and wisdom. Sometimes, just in stopping, one discovers the capacity for awareness and wakefulness in one's life for the very first time.

Between 1979 and this year, 2005, over sixteen thousand medical patients completed the MBSR program at the Stress Reduction Clinic at the University of Massachusetts Medical Center. The clinic takes the form of an eight-week course. People come to the hospital once a week for a class with twenty-five or thirty other people. In the sixth week there is an all-day silent retreat. We use audio recordings to guide people in various meditations. It's a well-defined, participatory curriculum that involves a lot of carefully guided meditation practice. The guidance is meant to give participants an understanding from the inside of what is being asked of them in terms of moment-to-moment, non-judgmental awareness and its embodiment both in formal practice and in daily living.

On another note, I've often wondered if you ever learned to ride a bicycle?

HH Dalai Lama: Yes.

Jon Kabat-Zinn: I ask because sometimes when we teach little children to ride a bicycle, it's not so easy for them to learn. But once you know how, you know for life. Sometimes children start with training wheels, which are gradually raised higher and then removed as they get the hang of it. In a sense, the guided meditations are like training wheels that you use until you learn how to cultivate mindfulness and mindful attention yourself. Going back to the bicycle analogy, you can then go on to train to become a Tour de France champion, or just ride the bike like an average person. That depends on your motivation.

As Ajahn Amaro was saying, meditation training often begins with paying attention to our breathing as an object of attention. However, in MBSR, as a skillful means, we often begin with eating, since people don't expect eating to be part of meditation training. It makes meditation practice much more ordinary and something of a surprise. Like breathing, eating is also very close to people's daily experience, yet it is freighted with major emotional issues for so many people. We all have the experience of eating, but usually we eat rather mindlessly. In MBSR, we start by eating one raisin very, very mindfully. We may take ten minutes, first smelling it, examining it visually, and feeling it in the hand, then tasting it and feeling the saliva in the mouth, and in this way cultivating awareness of an object that is very familiar to us, but that we are not usually very intimate with. People often say they have never really tasted a raisin before experiencing this example of mindful eating. It's a key discovery: If we pay attention, the world opens up. It lights up in new dimensions of experience.

After the raisin meditation, we then proceed to direct that same quality of attention to other aspects of our moment-to-moment experience —breathing, body sensations, hearing sounds, all sorts of perceptions of the eyes, ears, nose, mouth, and body—and then to the whole domain of thoughts and emotions. Thus we cultivate intimacy with the spaciousness of awareness, an awareness that can hold any or all objects of attention, and then bring that awareness into everyday life. Thus the true meditation practice becomes how you live your life, not how well you sit on a cushion. What we are really talking about is awareness. The various objects that we can pay attention to and be aware of are important, but most important is the attending itself, awareness itself, or mindfulness.

Dialogue and inquiry play a large role in every class. We talk together about our lives and, in particular, about how the meditation practice is developing from week to week. We may also, at times, judiciously recite poetry in the classroom to help ignite passion in the participants for certain mental and emotional qualities or feelings—a process that I later learned Thupten Jinpa calls "moistening the heart." A good poem often goes straight to the heart of a matter and can articulate in words things that are difficult to express any other way. MBSR also includes a range of formal meditation practices that people practice at home: a body scan done lying down on one's back, sitting meditation, mindful hatha yoga, and walking meditation.

There is a strong attitudinal and ethical foundation to MBSR. We don't give lectures on ethics and morality, but we are committed to embodying these qualities as best we can. Our intention is to create a container right there in the classroom for recognizing the beauty of other people and their integrity and dignity as human beings; for kindness and compassion; for a sense of gratitude for being alive, even with all of one's difficulties and dukkha; for cultivating interest and curiosity, and an orientation of non-striving. Americans are very driven people, always wanting to get someplace else. Learning meditation requires not trying to get someplace else so much as being where you already are, thus non-striving. It requires patience and being non-judgmental, being willing to have a beginner's mind that sees things freshly.

These are the kinds of things that we teach and the environment we create in the classroom and in the heart. Ajahn Amaro gave the vivid example of experiencing pain in one's knee. A lot of people who have chronic pain problems are referred to us. When you invite most people to pay attention to their pain, they don't say, "Wonderful! Why didn't I think of that before?" They say, "I don't want to pay attention to my pain; I want you to take it away" or "I want to get away from my pain, to escape, to distract myself." And we say, "Yes, but has that worked in the past? Just as an experiment, can you perhaps put a single toe in the water? Can you feel just the sensory element of the sensations you're calling pain, even for one moment?" Often, one discovers that there is also a whole universe of thinking around the sensations: "I hate this. This is killing me. How long is it going to last? My whole life is destroyed." All of those statements are merely thoughts, but people relate to them as if they are the truth about themselves and their immediate condition.

Then there is the whole emotional component to pain: anger, frustration, irritability, not liking one's body, feeling betrayed. When you hold these emotions in awareness without judging them so much, it pulls out the second arrow. It also releases you from shooting more arrows into yourself. You learn to cultivate a certain kind of equanimity in the face of discomfort. When you hear yourself saying, "This is killing me," you might ask instead, "In this moment, is this killing me?" The answer may very well be "No, but what about the next moment?" But remember, with mindfulness, we are trying to stay in *this* moment. We'll deal with the next moment in the next moment. In that way, we learn to *respond* more mindfully to any kind of stressful situation rather than *react* in a highly conditioned, mindless, automatic way. Bodily discomfort is just one example.

Out of this practice, over time, moments can emerge where you actually experience freedom and peace, right here in your own body, in your own mind, in your own life. People who claim they are no good at meditating can have a taste of this kind of thing if we make it interesting enough and create a safe enough container. They taste what's possible through practice and direct experience of the domain of being. And this is equally true, as Ajahn Amaro pointed out, for psychological suffering. You begin to see that there is value in attending to thoughts, emotions, and impulses, and even in monitoring the quality of awareness itself, as well as just sensations. A new dimension of being and knowing opens up in this discovery, a new way to inhabit your life, which is more balanced and less self-oriented. You begin to see that it's not just about "me": *my* pain, *my* anger, *my* frustration. The "my" is extra. Who is actually in pain? In the MBSR program, people spontaneously have experiences of no longer identifying so strongly with their mind states or their body states. This is a form of openness, of freedom. Here's one example, from a truck driver who came to the clinic with a chronic pain condition. He said:

> No, the pain is not gone. It's still here, but you know, when I start feeling it too much, I just sit aside somewhere, take ten, fifteen, twenty minutes, do my meditation, and that seems to take over. And if I can stay at least, say fifteen or thirty minutes or better, I can walk away and not even think about it for maybe three, four, five, six hours, maybe the whole day, depending on the weather.

The potential effect of this training on any pain condition, whether physical or emotional, or other medical conditions, requires an engagement with the experience itself. Usually we hold back; we don't want to be part of the experience. In mindfulness training we get in touch. We turn *toward* what is most aversive rather than *away* from it. We come to our senses, so to speak, literally and metaphorically. And as a consequence, a changed relationship to the experience, and to the suffering if pain is a part of it, usually arises.

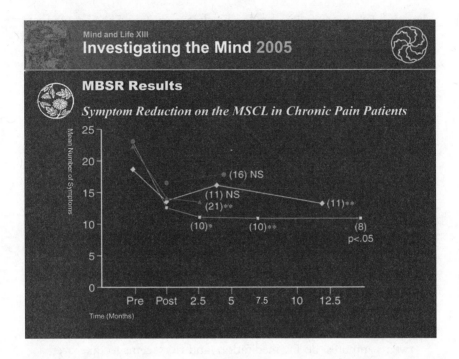

Figure 2. Mean symptom number as a function of time before and after MBSR and at follow-up times up to one year. MSCL stands for Medical Symptom Checklist. NS = not significant; p = probability of being random; * = p = .01; ** = p = .003.[17]

So now we come to the question of whether mindfulness actually influences the physiological or pathological nature of the pain itself. We did a study that showed reductions, over the course of eight weeks of training, of medical symptoms in patients who had chronic pain for a long time with no symptom relief.[16] The effect of MBSR training over eight weeks lasted for up to a year.[17] In other follow-up studies, it has lasted up to four years.[18] Of course, that is exactly what one hopes for: that a short initial exposure to meditation practice through MBSR translates into acting with greater wisdom and self-compassion, with love, you might say, and that you continue to practice and benefit, even in the face of pain and dukkha, for the rest of your life. It becomes so much a part of people's lives that they sometimes say, "At the beginning, I thought I was practicing meditation. Now it feels more like the meditation is practicing me."

To echo Matthieu and Ajahn Amaro, meditation is not merely a relaxation technique. It is not a technique at all, but a way of being and of seeing, resting on a foundation of deep inquiry into the nature of self, and offering the potential for liberation from the small-mindedness of self-preoccupation. Often people will say after a few weeks in the program, "What a minute! This isn't stress reduction; this is my whole life!" It is a moment of revelation.

Since about 1990, MBSR programs have spread, first slowly, then more rapidly, across the United States, Canada, and around the world. There is now a large global community of professionals who do this kind of work in hospitals, clinics, and other environments. Many mindfulness-based interventions modeled on MBSR have sprung up. For example, you'll be hearing from both Zindel Segal and John Teasdale about mindfulness-based cognitive therapy, or MBCT.

On another axis related to the work of MBSR, our cohosts from Johns Hopkins and Georgetown University Medical Center are now deeply engaged in the new field called integrative medicine, teaching the principles of mind/body medicine to medical students and the house staff, as well as delivering integrative care to medical patients. There are now twenty-nine medical schools,[19] many of them represented here today, that are part of the Consortium of Academic Health Centers for Integrative Medicine. I think it's fair to say that mindfulness is a core element of their mission. Integrative medicine is a new discipline within medicine that is helping to bring mindfulness-based interventions into the mainstream, along with other compelling evidence-based ways of restoring medicine to both its Hippocratic roots and its promise in the twenty-first century. This is a very positive development in restructuring health care and medicine, and for putting the "care" back into "health care."

In my final few moments, I'll just mention two studies. Richard Davidson will talk about the second one, which we did in collaboration. It is a small randomized trial of MBSR that we conducted in a corporate work setting to investigate how the brain and immune system change as people regulate emotion when they're under work stress or life stress.[20] As you will see, we obtained some exciting and promising results.

The study I will present now looked at whether meditation can influence the healing process in psoriasis, a skin disease that is an uncontrolled cell proliferation of the epidermis, the growing layer of the skin.[21] Psoriasis can cover the whole body, and stress makes it much worse. It flares up under high emotional stress, and it tends to go away when you're not under stress. The ultraviolet light in sunlight is very good for it, so in northern climates, the treatment for psoriasis is ultraviolet phototherapy. Patients stand in a light box, naked, so their skin is exposed, but their head and eyes are shielded. Patients come three times a week for up to four months, and gradually their skin clears.

It's not like a day at the beach, but more like being cooked in a toaster oven. The original idea for the study was that, since these patients were standing there naked, being exposed to ultraviolet light under very stressful conditions, perhaps it would be useful to guide them in mindfulness meditation while they were undergoing their treatments. Perhaps they would develop greater equanimity and be less stressed, and drop out of treatment less frequently. Then it occurred to us that perhaps it might be a good experimental protocol for asking an even deeper question: Can the mind itself influence the rate of healing, on top of the effect of the UV light? To tip the scale in that direction, as the guided meditation sequence unfolded we included a visualization of the UV light slowing down the rapidly growing cells in the epidermis.

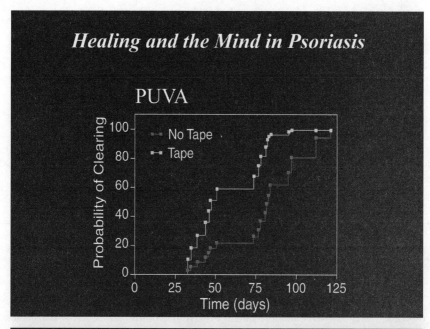

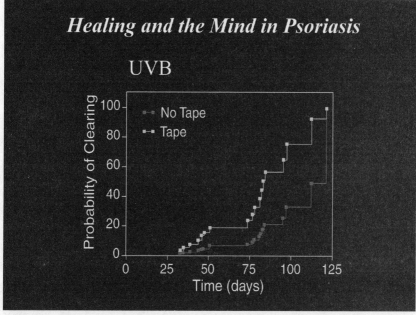

Figure 3. Estimated probability of skin clearing as a function of time for subjects in the guided meditation condition (Tape) and the control condition (No Tape). PUVA = photochemotherapy with UVA; UVB = phototherapy in the B wavelength region.[22]

We did this study twice, because the first time we didn't believe the results.[23] The patients are not in the light box for very long each time—a few minutes, increasing to maybe fifteen minutes by the end. We found that the meditators healed at a much faster rate than the nonmeditators. All other conditions were the same. The statistical analysis showed them healing at approximately four times the rate of those who were receiving the light treatments but were not meditating.

The implication is that something going on in the mind is strongly influencing the healing process at the level of the skin. It must be working all the way down to the level of the gene expression that controls cell replication. It could be influencing it through the nervous system, the endocrine system, the immune system, inflammatory responses, or a combination of these—we don't know the mechanism. Psoriasis is not skin cancer, but it shares some of the same genes with skin cancer, so this study has some interesting implications for cancer treatment. It was also a cost-effectiveness study, in that faster skin clearing means fewer treatments and less cost. It is also an example of integrative medicine, since the meditative intervention is integrated into the delivery of the allopathic treatment.

In summary, mindfulness-based interventions like MBSR and its relatives are an attempt to introduce core Buddhist meditative practices and principles into medicine and psychiatry in a universal framework that is still as true as possible to the dharma, thereby expanding the range of medical and psychological models for understanding disease and for approaching people suffering from chronic diseases and stress-related conditions with greater compassion and wisdom.

In medicine, the Hippocratic oath expresses a sacred relationship between the doctor and the patient. But it can't be a sacred relationship if the doctor is so busy and stressed that he or she is not really present and listening. So we now train medical students to be more mindful and heartful during patient encounters.

We all agree that the science of the mind/body connection is in its infancy. Nevertheless, promising findings have been reported over many years, and they are beginning to influence and expand interest in a number of areas in science and medicine. You will be hearing more about these in some of the presentations to follow, along with discussions of possible pathways and mechanisms of action.

To conclude, I want to say that the work I have presented was done and continues to be done by a number of people at University of Massachusetts, a kind of sangha whose members have all been very dedicated to dharma practice over many decades. Dr. Saki Santorelli, who now leads the Center for Mindfulness and the Stress Reduction Clinic, is in the audience, as are a number of other colleagues who teach there now or have taught there in the past.

I very much welcome this conversation among scientists, clinicians, and contemplative practitioners from many different lineages, so that we can ask deep questions about how to best serve people who are suffering, whether in hospitals, in schools, in government or politics, or in prisons. Human beings being human beings, the possibilities we're discussing here have tremendous potential for becoming a reality.

Matthieu Ricard: The presentations from Ajahn Amaro and Jon Kabat-Zinn have made it clear that meditation can be integrated into our everyday lives in a variety of ways. It is practical and fundamental, not some exotic practice. We've seen some of what meditation can do to improve the quality of our experience, but what is the correlation between long-term practice and changes in our brain? Also, what about different types of meditation: one-pointed attention, generating compassion, being in an open presence of awareness? How are these reflected in lasting changes in the brain? What can we study about that? This is what Richard Davidson is going to explain to us.

RICHARD DAVIDSON *Mind-Brain-Body Interaction and Meditation*

Many peripheral biological systems exist within a network of neural and endocrine connections that mediate the influence of the brain on peripheral biological function. Connections from the body to the brain are reciprocated in most of these systems. This anatomical and functional arrangement permits the mind to influence the body and vice versa. Meditation is a form of mental training that involves the voluntary alteration of patterns of neural activity and can have effects on peripheral biology through these mechanisms. This presentation offers

47

examples from recent and ongoing studies of the neural, immune, and endocrine changes produced by meditation to illustrate possible mechanisms by which meditation can promote increased mental and physical health.

Your Holiness, it's wonderful to be back with you. We're so grateful for the time you spend with us and, most importantly, the inspiration to do this work.

I will focus on three big points today. The first is that people differ in how inherently happy they are—their trait levels of happiness—and other virtuous characteristics such as compassion. The second point is that humans' capacity to regulate their emotions plays a key role in modulating differences among people in how happy, resilient, or compassionate they are. The third point, which is really at the intersection of our respective traditions, is that happiness and compassion can be regarded as the product of skills that mental training can enhance.

Most people are poor at predicting what will make them happy. Scientists have found differences among people in what they refer to as a happiness "set point." These differences among individuals are associated with different patterns of brain function and peripheral biology.

However, humans are endowed with the capacity to voluntarily regulate their emotions, and there is evidence to suggest that this competence can be learned. I emphasize the importance of mental training, which involves thinking about happiness and compassion not just as traits but as skills. If they are skills, that implies that the mind and the brain can be transformed in ways that will also affect the body. This will be the substance of my comments today.

I want to begin by reminding everyone that in addition to being a state and a trait, in our country happiness, or at least its pursuit, is also an unalienable right.

HH Dalai Lama: Not only in America.

Richard Davidson: In fact, I think there are many countries that take this right more seriously than we do. Just to remind everyone, our Declaration of Independence states, "We hold these truths to be self-evident, that all men are created equal, that they are endowed by their Creator with certain unalienable rights; that among these are life, liberty and the pursuit of happiness." It's our conviction, Your Holiness, that our interactions with you have underscored the importance of this pursuit and the fact that our culture has not taken this sufficiently seriously. We think the scientific research will be helpful in showing that these skills really can be learned.

The first issue I'd like to turn to is, How malleable are happiness and well-being? Do social and economic conditions modify our levels of happiness? And what do the answers to these questions imply about happiness?

A study was conducted that collected data from tens of thousands of people using surveys.[24] One question we examined is whether marriage can buy you happiness. The data show that there is an elevation in happiness when people get married, but remarkably, after just a few years, people return to their baseline. Five years later, people are actually lower than when they began.

I've been happily married for a long time, so it doesn't apply to everybody.

The next question is whether widowhood produces unhappiness. At the time of widowhood, we see a big decline in happiness, but remarkably it eventually comes back to what appears to be a set point. Again, these are real data—I'm not making this up.

The third question is one that our culture is particularly obsessed with: whether money can buy you happiness. If we look at the gross domestic product of the United States over a fifty-year period in relation to the percentage of people who report themselves to be very happy, the gross domestic product rises, showing a very strong economy, but the percentage of people who report themselves very happy is essentially flat and even goes slightly down. It doesn't matter what indicator of happiness you use, they all show the same effect.

What do all of these findings imply? Can happiness be enhanced, or are we all stuck at our set points? What are the underlying brain mechanisms, and how might they influence the body? Can we change the brain through mental training, and thereby influence the mind and the body in beneficial ways?

Most scientists accept the notion that emotion is governed by a distributed neural circuitry. Different parts of the brain work together, including cortical and subcortical components. The cortex is the most developed part of the brain over the course of evolution, and while it has historically been thought to mostly play a role in perception and thinking, modern research clearly indicates that it also plays a crucial role in emotion. Subcortical areas such as the amygdala and ventral striatum also play important roles and are interconnected with cortical regions, particularly in the prefrontal cortex. These circuits of emotion have bidirectional communication with the body, including the autonomic nervous system, the endocrine system, and the immune system. This indicates that when we change the brain, we inevitably influence the body. Correspondingly, when the body changes, it in turn influences the brain.

Your Holiness, when we were together in Dharamsala at the 2004 Mind and Life meeting on neuroplasticity, we talked about how the brain can change in response to experience and training. There is good evidence to show that musical training can influence the brain very substantially.[25] Learning new motor skills, such as juggling, can influence the brain.[26] Michael Meaney showed us, in his presentation in Dharamsala, that how a mother behaves toward her offspring dramatically affects their brains.[27] We also know that neurogenesis, which is the growth of new neurons in the brain, can be impaired by stress and that exercise can promote neurogenesis. Some new evidence from our lab suggests that training in emotion regulation may also influence the functional activity of the brain.[28]

In one study, we showed people a picture of a baby with a facial tumor and asked them to wish that this baby would be healed and free from suffering.[29] It turns out that when people adopt that attitude, it changes their brain. The part of the brain called the amygdala, which is important in detecting threat and negative emotion especially, is modulated when people transform their emotion to make it more positive and to express compassion.

People differ in how skilled they are at voluntarily regulating their emotions. Those who are better able to regulate their negative emotions show less activation in the amygdala and more activation in an area called the ventromedial prefrontal cortex, which is involved in emotion regulation and decision making.

We also found a connection between the endocrine system and how well people can regulate their negative emotions. If we look at the average curve for a normal daily change in cortisol, a hormone that plays a key role in response to stress, we see elevated levels of cortisol in the morning.

They go down throughout the day and are at their lowest point in the evening before we go to bed.

HH Dalai Lama: What is the reason that the cortisol level is generally higher in the morning and goes down in the evening?

Richard Davidson: That's an excellent question. It has to do with regulating body temperature and other characteristics of our bodies. There are certain energetic things in the morning that the elevation in cortisol helps to promote.

Looking at different people, we see a lot of variation in individual patterns of daily cortisol levels. Some people have less of a reduction of cortisol at the end of the day. It turns out that it's a problem if cortisol levels aren't reduced in the evening. The more they're reduced in the evening, the better the health outcomes that appear to be associated.

We found that people who are good at regulating their emotions, and specifically at transforming negative emotions, have a better profile of cortisol levels, with a steeper decline at the end of the day. In particular, people who show more activation in the ventromedial prefrontal cortex while regulating negative emotions also have lower levels of cortisol at the end of the day.

A very general hypothesis is that some forms of meditation strengthen the cortical regulatory circuitry in the brain that in turn modulates the dynamics of subcortical emotional reactivity. In our work with long-term Buddhist meditation practitioners,[30] we found that meditation is associated with marked increases in the brain's electrical signs of activation expressed in the fast-frequency oscillation known as gamma, particularly in the prefrontal cortex, which is important for aspects of regulating emotion. This is consistent with the idea that meditation is not simple relaxation. We also see an increased synchrony between the prefrontal cortex and other regions of the brain in long-term practitioners. This idea of synchrony was pioneered by Wolf Singer, who will be speaking this afternoon, and also was championed by Francisco Varela in his work.

The increases in the gamma frequency are much greater in long-term practitioners than in control subjects who recently learned to do the same meditation practice and had been meditating for just one week before we tested them.

There is also a very striking association between the clarity or luminosity that practitioners report during the compassion meditation and the magnitude of the gamma signal. We asked the practitioner to push a button to indicate the intensity of perceived clarity every time there was a change in the subjective experience of clarity. One thing that's very striking to me as a scientist is that untrained individuals are not very good at reporting on the qualities of their mind, whereas the long-term practitioners we work with have a greater facility to report more accurately on subjective experience. The association between reports and brain signals among long-term practitioners may therefore actually be stronger, because their reports of experience are more refined. The signal in the brain that's associated with these reports of clarity is specifically concentrated in the prefrontal cortex.

In the laboratory, we've taken a very simple approach where we have practitioners meditate for short periods of time. We alternate those periods of meditation with a neutral state so that we can contrast the changes in the brain during both states. So far we have analyzed data on eleven long-term practitioners and twelve age-matched controls who were novice meditators. All the controls were individuals who were interested in meditating, and they were taught the same compassion practices done by the long-term practitioners. This is how Matthieu described to me the meditation the participants were doing:

> Here, what we have tried to do, for the sake of the experiment, is to generate a state in which love and compassion permeate the whole mind, with no other consideration, reasoning, or discursive thoughts. This is sometimes called pure compassion, or nonreferential compassion (in the sense that it does not focus on particular objects to arouse love or compassion), or all-pervading compassion.

When we used functional magnetic resonance imaging to look at the brain while people were doing this meditation, there were some remarkable findings. Many areas of the brain were more activated during compassion meditation as compared to the neutral state.

We found that compassion meditation changes the brain's response to the presentation of distressing sounds. When we present a recording of a woman screaming for just a couple of seconds, the practitioners show a remarkable increase in activation in the insula. The insula is a part of the brain critical for communicating with the body and provides information on the state of the body to the rest of the brain. Different visceral organs project information to the insula. The insula has been implicated in empathy. Another brain region, the medial prefrontal cortex, has been implicated in self-relevant processing. This area of the brain gets activated when people think about themselves. For example, if you suggest an adjective and ask people whether this adjective describes them, that area of the brain becomes very active. This area of the brain associated with the self is deactivated when people are generating compassion, which is very much a selfless state.

The last question I'd like to turn to is whether these differences are actually results of training. A skeptic might say that maybe these long-term practitioners were that way to start with. In science we always have to entertain the skeptics. One finding that speaks to this question is the relation with length of practice. The longer the person has practiced, the stronger many of these effects are.

A second finding comes from the randomized controlled trial we did with Jon Kabat-Zinn, which he mentioned earlier.[31] The question was whether beneficial effects can be achieved with the kind of short-term training in mindfulness-based stress reduction that Jon talked about. We randomized novices either to receive the meditation intervention or to be part of a control group that waited for two months before receiving the training.

Testing showed an increase in left prefrontal activity in the brain among those who had done the meditation training. The control group actually showed an increase in activity on the right side of the prefrontal cortex.

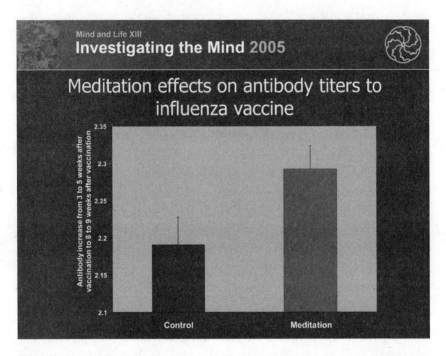

Figure 4. Antibody titers in response to influenza vaccine in meditators who completed an MBSR course and wait-list controls.[32]

We also gave the entire group an ordinary flu vaccine and then looked at the amounts of antibodies produced in response to the vaccine to give us an idea of how well their immune systems were functioning. The meditation group showed a bigger increase in the amount of antibodies produced in response to the vaccine compared to the control group.

To summarize and conclude, external factors have only limited effects on our level of happiness. People differ in their emotional dispositions. Although these affective styles are relatively stable, we believe they can be changed. Profiles of brain function associated with positive emotional traits are also associated with downstream effects on the endocrine and immune systems that might promote certain kinds of physical health. Finally, meditation has demonstrable effects on the brain and may represent one of the few ways in which purely mental training has been demonstrated to have a robust impact on brain function.

I'd like to close with a quote from Albert Einstein:[33]

A human being is a part of the whole, called by us "Universe," a part limited in time and space. He experiences himself, his thoughts and feelings, as something separated from the rest—a kind of optical delusion of his consciousness. This delusion is a kind of prison for us, restricting us to our personal desires and to affection for a few persons nearest to us. Our task must be to free ourselves from this prison by widening our circle of compassion to embrace all living creatures and the whole of nature in its beauty. Nobody is able to achieve this completely, but the striving for such achievement is in itself a part of the liberation and a foundation for inner security.

I'd like to express my deep bow of gratitude to Francisco, and also to Antoine Lutz, who is in the audience. Antoine, you should stand, because you have been so directly responsible for so much of this work. I also want to acknowledge the many other members of my lab who have contributed to this work.

SESSION 1 DIALOGUE

In addition to HH Dalai Lama and the presenters, translators, and · moderator, panelists for this session include Father Thomas Keating and Sharon Salzberg.

Matthieu Ricard: The different points that have been raised in this morning's session can show us that meditation is not simply a hobby or a way we choose to kill time, but has a really deep effect on our well-being through the way we deal with the inner conditions of happiness, as opposed to trying desperately to control outer conditions.

We would like to ask His Holiness to comment on what has been said this morning, and we will enter into this with a few questions from Jon.

Jon Kabat-Zinn: The first question I have, your Holiness, is this: Have any specific meditation practices been successfully used in the Tibetan medical tradition for particular medical ailments or mental afflictions?

HH Dalai Lama: I don't know. My physicians never taught me any meditation. Of course, there might be some situations where a physician teaches a specific form of mental training to patients.

Jon Kabat-Zinn: The second question is whether the experience of pure awareness is itself physically or mentally healing.

HH Dalai Lama: This is a slightly complex issue. When you experience what the Buddhist language describes as an uncontrived state of mind, or pure awareness, in that instance the attention is diverted from any emotional or physical pain you might normally have. In that state of awareness, the mind is distracted, so at that moment there may be a form of healing or an experience of freedom. But the question is, When you get out of that state, will the pain come back? Maybe. So here, it's a form of a diversion, or it might act as a tranquilizer.

On the other hand, if you really focus on the pain or the suffering itself, this might have a different effect. For example, if your approach is based on the recognition of the dukkha condition of your existence, and the recognition also that the experience of pain itself is transient and subject to change, this might actually have a much more positive effect. Similarly, as some of the speakers mentioned, the degree of one's self-identification with the pain and the grasping that goes with that might make a difference in the intensity of the pain. For example, one of the characteristics of compassion is that it immediately opens your heart outward to a much more expansive field. That in itself will have an effect, releasing this grasping of one's self-centered focus.

What Einstein said, as Richie quoted, is definitely true. If we find some way to get out of this prison of self-centeredness and reach out to the wider common humanity, truly this will have an impact.

Jon Kabat-Zinn: Thank you, Your Holiness. My third question is, Can we make a valid distinction between Buddhadharma on the one hand, and universal dharma on the other?[34] Or are they fundamentally the same regarding the cultivation of awareness, compassion, and wisdom?

HH Dalai Lama: The importance of these positive emotions or qualities applies to all spiritual traditions. We are trying to promote universal spiritual values with help from scientists. Part of what we are doing here is finding ways in which we can reinforce the values that have been taught by the great spiritual traditions over thousands of years. These are common human values.

Matthieu Ricard: It seems very appropriate at this point to request Father Keating to share a few thoughts from another great contemplative tradition. How do you see the pursuit of contemplation, especially in terms of helping altruistic love and unconditional compassion become not just second nature, but our true nature?

Father Keating: It seems to me that I've heard three different issues discussed here this morning. First of all, it's been emphasized that the Mind and Life Institute is creating something that has never happened before, namely a sincere and serious dialogue between the scientific community, or at least part of it, and religion. This institute has been fostered by His Holiness himself, so I want to thank you, Your Holiness, for your initiative in starting a dialogue that is enormously important. I've been engaged in Buddhist-Christian dialogue for many years, and it feels wonderful to be able to extend the dialogue to other intelligent, if not religious, human beings in the scientific community. They will find that mystics are not so stupid after all. I'm sure we will experience that scientists are on the spiritual journey too, whether they realize it or not. Just to be born is to be on the spiritual journey.

The second point is the issue of meditation as described in Jon's presentation, which was so wonderful. Buddhist meditation emphasizes clarity of mind: mindfulness. This would be very suitable for initiating beginners and for bringing people into the experiential aspect of spiritual practice if it could be abstracted from belief systems. What we're talking about here is not just religions or external practice, but the spirituality of religions, which is something else. I think it's the interior practice of religion or spirituality that affects health and produces the effects you're beginning to see in the brain. So we feel completely at one with our Buddhist brothers and sisters and, indeed, all the other spiritual traditions of the world. We hope these discussions can bring those values into the experience of oneness that is so essential for the globalization process and its contribution to world peace. The new physics, for instance, is saying things that are more mystical than you'll ever hear in a Sunday sermon. I've heard one physicist quoted as saying that you can't have a thought without influencing the rest of the universe—instantaneously! Maybe it's a small influence, but the idea suggests an extraordinary interconnectedness or interdependence of everything in creation. This has enormous effects on religions and science, including how we see each other and the rest of the world.

The third point relates to what we heard about the physiognomy of the experience of contemplative prayer as looked at from inside the brain. It would be fun to see what contemplatives think about these results. Instead of you experimenting with us, how about letting us experiment with you? Let's see if your findings correspond to our experience. In other words, this is the beginning of taking interior or mystical experience seriously. I think this knowledge that goes beyond the discursive, or analytical, and takes seriously the intuitive capacities of the brain—what in religious circles we call the human soul or human spirit—will be a great contribution to the development of knowledge in all its aspects.

So it seems to me that, thanks to the initiatives of the Mind and Life Institute and His Holiness, we're on the verge of a giant leap in the way human beings understand themselves, and in our accountability or stewardship for the rest of creation. Our own health or transformation is the beginning of that process.

Matthieu Ricard: Sharon, you have been practicing and teaching not only insight, or mindfulness, meditation, but also metta, the cultivation of loving-kindness and compassion, accessed by identifying that aspiration for well-being in ourselves as a way to become more open to others. How do you feel this element of practice is integrated with all that has been said?

Sharon Salzberg: First, I was struck when Richie said that a part of the brain seems to reflect a sense of self. I wondered, does the hardware exist so that one could be measured all day long to see how often that part of the brain lights up? It would be shocking, probably.

Going back to the first thing Ajahn Amaro said, the concepts and ideas that have been presented here are not dogma. They are not to be taken as blind belief, but to be put into practice so we can see for ourselves if they are true. I've always found that to be a breathtaking vision of human potential: that we can understand, if we are willing to look for ourselves, that we are not stuck in any way. I found that be to one of the most powerful comments.

Ajahn Amaro also spoke about the different kinds of suffering: natural suffering, or pain, and superimposed, or adventitious, suffering. I think sometimes the first kind of suffering is devastating. It can be just outrageous. What is called for at that time may be a whole other means of restoring balance or a sense of healing. But many times, for most of us, that distinction between the pain and what we make of it is critical. To know the difference is not only the essence of spiritual life in some way, but also the difference between loss and despair, between an ordeal and hopelessness, or between an unfortunate circumstance and bitterness. That is a tremendous distinction to be made. I see practices like mindfulness and loving-kindness coming into play right there, because we are capable of so much, and not only for ourselves, but in relationship to others as well. People often think of meditation as leading to passivity, just being complacent or easygoing. If we can address that superimposed suffering somewhat, we will have more energy to look at the direct experience of the pain or the circumstance and try to find a way to be in a new relationship with it, for ourselves and for others.

I have one question, which came from looking at Richie's photo of the baby with the growth. It was so difficult to look at. I wonder if the ways we treat, or are trained to see, our own suffering affect how we see the suffering of others. It makes sense in terms of common sense or logic. If we are habituated to fear, denial, disgust, or condemnation instead of kindness, it makes sense that this is how we would view the suffering and distress of others. I wonder if any research has been done on those correlations.

Richard Davidson: It's an interesting question. There's some evidence to indicate that the personality of the perceiver influences the way he or she interprets and responds to an emotional picture of that sort. But research hasn't specifically focused on your question, which is the extent to which people's attitude of kindness toward themselves affects how they react to such pictures or encounters in the world.

Matthieu Ricard: Some studies also show that there are two basic patterns of altruism. One is centered on oneself: We feel distress when facing others' suffering and we cannot stand that, so we want to do something to relieve that distress. Genuine altruism is not just about that. It's a deep concern for others that may indeed be reflected in a reduction in activation of brain regions related to the self.

Alan Wallace: Richie, my attention was also caught, as Sharon's was, when you spoke of the part of the brain associated with the self, and how it's deactivated when compassion arises. I'd love to bring a bit more clarity to this, for my own sake. Exactly what are you referring to when you say "the self"? I'd like to suggest three possibilities. One is the self that, in the Cartesian mode, stands apart from the body and mind, the unmoved mover that governs and regulates the body and mind. This is completely refuted in Buddhism. Have we found the neural correlate of a Cartesian self?

A second possibility is the sense of personal identity that we all have. You have a sense that I'm speaking to you; I have a sense that you're responding to me right now. Somebody calls my name and I say, "Yes, what can I do for you?" That sense of personal identity certainly exists. Is that the self of these neural correlates?

The third possibility is what Buddhists call self-cherishing, self-centeredness, or simply, in the vernacular, selfishness: "My well-being is most important, so look out! I need to get things for me!" That's not equivalent to either of the other two. For which one of those have you found a correlate?

Richard Davidson: It's really for none of them. When people are given an adjective, such as "cheerful," and are asked whether that adjective is characteristic of themselves, a very complex process begins, which we don't really understand in detail. It begins with assessing whether aspects that they consider part of who they are, are in fact reflected in this adjective. The experiment shows that when you ask people whether adjectives of that sort are characteristic of themselves, the medial cortex tends to become activated. If you ask whether the adjective is characteristic of your friend John, it doesn't get activated, though it's doing the same work with the same stimulus. So it's activated by something in this process when the mind, or at least an untrained mind, introspects about its self-image.

Alan Wallace: So it's not the Cartesian self, and not selfishness, but who you think you are, your sense of personal identity.

Richard Davidson: Yes, it's most closely related to that.

Father Keating: I'd like to know what part silence plays in your research on mental training. Do you have any data on what the brain looks like when it's completely silent of thought?

Richard Davidson: I will ask Matthieu to comment on silence, since he has been a very important collaborator and research participant, and has had training that most of us have not had.

Matthieu Ricard: Well, silence in what sense? Does silence mean the absence of discursive thinking—the mental chatter that's always taking place as we are engaged in reasoning, interpreting the outer world, ruminating on the past, or imagining the future? Of course, that chain reaction of thoughts can have an obscuring aspect when it happens automatically. Silencing this rumination and mental construction can be a meditative state. Somehow we find an enhanced awareness of clarity and stability behind the stream or veil of thoughts and their content. This is by no means silence in the sense of dullness, drowsiness, darkness, or obscurity. It's a very vivid, aware state of mind. You could call it silence of the mental constructions, but it is in no way a silence of awareness. That is how the practitioner would perceive these states.

Father Keating: From the perspective of Christian meditation, which we usually call contemplation—the two words are interchangeable at this level of discussion—we emphasize the intentionality of silence. That is to say, silence as an intention has a significant effect on the process of meditation, whether you're experiencing thoughts, feelings, external sounds, or whatever. Getting used to disregarding the flow of thought leads into deeper levels of interior silence and peace. At that level we seem to be touching or experiencing a deeper aspect of human nature than ordinary psychological awareness. This is usually known as the spiritual level of our being or, in terms of the perennial philosophy, the intuitive level of consciousness and beyond. The mental training that you've started to do in these various units around the country, which is a wonderful contribution toward alleviating people's suffering, might be enhanced by the introduction of the aspect of intentionality, which enables one to deliberately let go of negative thoughts or feelings.

Christian meditation also emphasizes heartfulness. In other words, there's a deliberate, affective movement of the spiritual will toward the ends that you are trying to achieve. St. John of the Cross puts it in terms of a relationship with God—God meaning the ultimate reality or whatever your label for the ultimate reality might be. God happens to be the Judeo-Christian way of expressing this mystery. It's a relationship with ultimate reality that constitutes human health, because the source of our being is also sustaining us at all times. Obviously, living according to our inner nature will produce health.

St. John of the Cross says human health consists primarily of being continuously in the presence of ultimate reality. That's a kind of "supermindfulness," in which we're mindful not just of the objects of the senses, which is a preliminary discipline, but of the broader reality out of which all sense experiences are emerging. Another way of describing it is awareness of the ground of our being. Relating to ultimate reality is the ultimate source of security, love, and freedom. It is who we really are, even if we don't realize it. Stop thinking often enough, and this begins to insinuate itself into activity and forms the background or a kind of fourth dimension to the three-dimensional world we live in. How to bring people into that space is the purpose of religion, and it could be the purpose of medicine.

Jon Kabat-Zinn: Your implication is very well taken. Attention and intention work beautifully together to further the possibility of waking up to the actuality of one's experience, which you could call the ground of being—or the groundlessness of being. There's no interruption, then, in the continuity of experience between the sensory domain and the domain of awareness itself, which is virtually boundless. That is exactly what Albert Einstein was pointing to in the quotation that Richie shared with us.

In MBSR, our orientation is that the silence you are speaking of is the domain of awareness itself. It is available in every moment. The question is whether we can tune the organism, through the skillful use of attention and intention, to cultivate the capacity to be more in touch, in every domain, with that underlying thunderous silence.

Matthieu Ricard: We have seen something of the long-term effects of meditation and even the change that an eight-week course can bring, but we obviously need to do more longitudinal studies, over months and years. I think Alan could say a few words about a project designed to engage in just such a longitudinal study.

Alan Wallace: Cliff Saron is in the audience. He is the principal scientific investigator of what we are calling the Shamatha Project. I recently learned that I have been named the principal contemplative investigator for the project—a new category. We're aiming to do a one-year longitudinal study of about thirty-two people living in a retreat setting and meditating eight to ten hours a day. The primary emphasis will be on training attention, developing greater clarity and stability of attention, together with the cultivation of the heart. I love the word "heartfulness." An absolutely crucial element of the training will be cultivating what Buddhists call the divine abidings, or the immeasurable qualities of loving-kindness, compassion, empathetic joy, and equanimity.

Our real aim is to develop a one-year project, but we will start a bit more modestly, with the first stage being a three-month research project with the highest standards of scientific rigor. We have a marvelous team at the University of California, Davis, and we're planning to start next September.[35]

Matthieu Ricard: It's a very exciting prospect.

Father Keating: That would certainly be a wonderful experiment. At the same time, I think the project that's immediately before us is how to introduce this in the ordinary stream of everyday living, for those who are suffering and want some help right away, wherever they are. I wonder if it might be useful to further clarify the distinction between pain and suffering. I've heard the words used interchangeably, and one definition that I thought was fairly insightful was that pain is just a normal part of life. It's an essential situation in a limited universe. Suffering is when you resist the pain. Jesus suggests in the gospel that it would be better not to do this when he says, "Resist not evil," meaning what you perceive as evil. Suffering is probably the thing we chiefly regard as evil, as well as death. So if our attitude toward pain were to be accepting it as it is, then useless suffering might be greatly diminished.

SESSION 2

POSSIBLE BIOLOGICAL SUBSTRATES OF MEDITATION

Modern scientific knowledge of how stress affects the brain and the body, and how the brain can become reorganized as a result of practices that strengthen attention and awareness and promote learning and adaptive ways of dealing with stress and change, has burgeoned over the past decade. This session, moderated by Richard Davidson, showcases some of the latest scientific research on these topics to provide a foundation for investigating the likely mechanisms and pathways through which meditation might exert its various effects. The elucidation of the biological substrates of stress and neuroplasticity offers a cogent framework for the design of new research that can extend and deepen this understanding.

Richard Davidson: Your Holiness, this afternoon we're going to consider possible biological underpinnings of meditation. We have two presenters who are world experts in different aspects of brain and biology. Wolf Singer has dedicated his scientific career to understanding how the network organization of the brain, in synchrony, gives rise to higher mental functions. That is the topic that he will be addressing.

WOLF SINGER *Synchronization of Brain Rhythms as a Possible Mechanism for the Unification of Distributed Mental Processes*

The brain is organized in a highly distributed way and lacks a convergence center for the coherent interpretation of the numerous parallel processes that occur simultaneously within functionally specialized regions. This raises the question of how subsystems are integrated so that their individual results can give rise to unified percepts. It is proposed that this integration is achieved at least in part by the synchronization of oscillatory activity in the beta and gamma frequency range. Beta and gamma frequency brain oscillations are fast rhythms that are associated with attention, perception, and learning. This interpretation is in accordance with neuronal activation patterns recorded during states of focused attention and meditation, since attentional processes serve binding functions, heighten awareness, and lead to the unification of distributed processes.

Your Holiness, it is a great honor for me to be here next to you, and to explain what we believe to be one of the neuronal substrates of the conscious states that characterize meditation. I will talk about the role of synchronous oscillatory activity in the brain, its relation to attention and consciousness, and some implications that it may have in explaining pathologies such as schizophrenia.

There is evidence that states of meditation are associated with the synchronization of oscillatory activity in a very high-frequency range in the cerebral cortex, the so-called gamma frequencies of around forty hertz. Under certain conditions, when the brain is appropriately activated, there are grouped discharges of neurons and an oscillatory patterning of this activity in the range of about forty hertz.

My colleagues and I discovered this phenomenon in Frankfurt about fifteen years ago,[36] and since then, we've pursued the idea that this signal might be required for the integration of distributed activity in the brain. We questioned whether there is something special about synchronized activity in the brain and discovered that there is: Synchronized activity has a much stronger impact on cells that receive this activity than temporally uncoordinated activity does. Therefore, synchronizing responses is equivalent to selecting responses for further processing.

Only synchronized responses profit from each other to become more effective, so synchronizing responses is equivalent to defining relations among the neurons that are synchronously active. In this way, it is possible to define relations among neuronal responses that are distributed across the brain. Precise synchronization of neuronal activity can, in principle, serve as a signature of relatedness in signal processing and, by virtue of this, also in learning. Synchrony defines which neurons cooperate in order to convey their message jointly.

Why should the signal of relatedness among distributed neuronal responses be such an important issue for the functioning of the brain? Our hypothesis relates to the fact that we in Western societies have a wrong intuition about how the brain is organized. We have a Cartesian view. We think that somewhere in the brain there ought to be a convergence center, a singular place where all the information comes together for a coherent interpretation of the world. This would be the place where decisions are reached, and also the place where the intentional self has its seat.

Modern brain research now describes a completely different picture of the organization of the human brain. Areas of the cerebral cortex are interconnected very intensively with one another, but there is no evidence for a convergence center or a pyramidal hierarchical organization. Different brain areas deal with very different inputs—from the eye, from the ear, and from the touch senses—and are also connected to areas belonging to the limbic system, which attach emotional connotations to the contents of conscious experience. There is no single place in the brain where an observer could be located, a command structure could be implemented, or the self could have its seat. It is a highly distributed system in which many functions occur simultaneously and there is no coordinator. They self-organize. In such a system, it becomes extremely important that the many neuronal responses that are generated all the time get labeled so it is clear at any one moment in time which neurons are actually collaborating. We need a code that defines relations.

Because of this distributed organization, an object is represented in the brain by many thousands of neurons that are active at the same time, distributed over different areas. If you see a barking dog and touch its fur, you have input from the touch sense, the eyes, and the ears, and they are all simultaneously processed in different areas of the cerebral cortex, never coming together at any singular place. Somehow, in this distributed network, the representation of a barking dog with silky fur emerges. So the intuition that a single center must exist is wrong. There is no coordinator, no observer, no seat of the self.

Even within one modality, like the visual system, there are about thirty different areas in the cerebral cortex that process different contents. Some are interested in texture, others in color, others in emotion, and others in certain aspects of shapes, and all of these aspects are extracted simultaneously.

When complex pictures are decoded, activity from many different places in the brain must be bound together in a meaningful way in order to give rise to the percept of one of these horses, for example. One has to bind together the right contours and segregate them from the contours of the background. That can be quite a challenge, as this image illustrates (see figure 5).

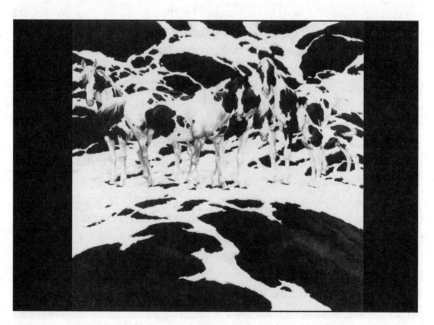

Figure 5. Example of the binding problem. In order to segregate the figures from the background and detect the horses, it is necessary to selectively bind the black and white surfaces belonging to individual horses and to segregate them from the black and white surfaces of the background.

Since there is no unique convergence center in the brain, representations of cognitive contents must consist of the coordinated activity of large numbers of neurons that may be distributed across many different areas of the cerebral cortex. This is why it is so important to define relations in such a distributed system. We need a code that defines with very high temporal precision, from instance to instance—because the contents of consciousness change very rapidly—which subset of the myriads of neurons actually contributes at any one moment in time to a coherent representation.

For the generation of distributed representations, neurons have to convey two messages in parallel. First, they have to signal through their activation whether the feature for which they are specialized is present. Second, they have to convey a message as to which other neurons they are cooperating with in this very moment to form a coherent representation. There is a lot of evidence now that the dynamic definition of relations is achieved by the synchronization of neuronal discharges and that this mechanism plays a key role in the coordination and integration of distributed brain processes.

In the scientific community, we are currently discussing a number of roles that this synchronization might play. (As a reminder, this synchronization is the same as the coherent oscillations that increase so dramatically when experienced practitioners engage in meditative states.) Possible roles include the simple function of perceptual grouping, which binds together features to get a coherent percept. There is evidence that synchronization is used by the brain to focus attention on certain inputs and make them more salient, or more effective. There is evidence that we self-generate these synchronous oscillatory patterns when we close our eyes and imagine something.[37] If we imagine a visual object, then the visual areas engage in this synchronous activity, which apparently reads out stored information.

We know that synchronous activity is very important for the integration of subsystems, as in the case of the barking dog, binding together the sound, the touch, and the image of the dog. Another function that is closely related to the focus of attention is the routing of activity through the extremely complex network of the brain. A big problem is that messages need to be sent from one place in the brain to another with high selectivity. How is this done when the connections are so intermingled? There is evidence that nature has found a way very much like when we use a radio to tune in to a transmitter. The sender and the receiver are in the same frequency, so they can resonate with a handshake, and then transmission of information becomes very selective.[38]

Synchronization is also involved in memory processes. In short-term memory, for example when you want to remember a telephone number or a few things for a short period of time, oscillations occur over the brain areas relevant for these processes. Synchronous activity is also used to inscribe long-term memories, because it is ideally suited to changing neuronal response properties in the long term.

I would like to give you a few selected examples of the involvement of synchrony in cognitive processes. An important feature is state dependency of response synchronization. Brains are not always in the same state. They may be drowsy and inattentive, or attentive. When one records an EEG from the scalp of a person in an attentive state, the brain waves have small amplitude and fairly high frequency. When the brain gets a bit drowsy and inattentive, large amplitude waves occur.[39]

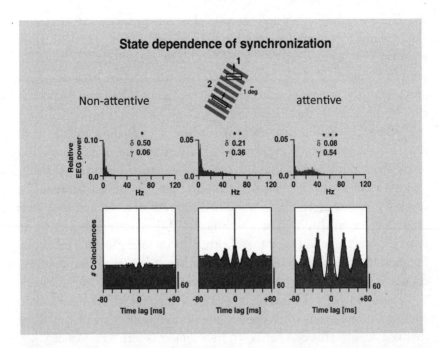

Figure 6. Two groups of neurons in the visual cortex of a cat were activated with a light stimulus (insert on top), and the amount of synchronization of the respective neuronal responses was assessed by computing cross-correlograms (bottom panels). At the same time, the frequency distribution of the ongoing electroencephalographic activity was measured (histograms in the middle). When the animal is in an attentive state (right panels), the electroencephalogram displays activity in the high-frequency range, and the neuronal responses are well synchronized, as indicated by the oscillatory modulation of the cross-correlogram (bottom right panel). As attention decreases (middle and left panels), low frequencies increase in the electroencephalogram, and the synchronization of the responses is reduced.

The interesting finding is that synchronous activity occurs only when the brain is in a highly attentive state. It disappears completely when the brain gets drowsy and inattentive. Even though the nerve cells respond very actively, as before, they are not temporally coordinated in their activity. So, rather than modulating the amount of activity, attention involves the coherence and synchronization of activity. This is an important issue. When the meditators go into this attentive state, they probably increase the coordination of distributed neuronal activity.

71

The same happens when an animal or an organism anticipates an action, when it prepares for something. A cat can be trained to distinguish a pattern that is presented on a screen and then respond quickly when the pattern changes. The cat knows when this will happen because a buzz announces the event. Researchers can then record the brain activity of these animals while they perform this act, and look for synchrony.

When the cat is not attentive—when it is feeding, which is its reward—the brain waves are slow, with no good synchrony among the different areas. But when a sound tells the animal to turn around immediately and react quickly to the changing pattern, then the activity between the cortical areas involved changes dramatically. All of a sudden, they start oscillating in synchrony. The cat produces this synchronous activity in anticipation that it will need these cortical areas to engage in a particular function. So the sender and receiver neurons tune in to the same frequency in order to allow better "handshaking."

There is also evidence that a critical amount of synchronization among neurons occurs when one becomes consciously aware of something that one sees.[40] This can be shown in a simple experiment. A noisy pattern that has no content is first presented to the subject. Then a word, in this case "cat," is presented, followed by another noisy, blurred pattern, and then a final word, either "cat" or "dog." Afterward, we ask the subjects whether they saw the first word and whether it was the same as the word shown at the end of the experiment.

There are three possible outcomes: The subject sees the first word, consciously remembers it, and recognizes whether it is the same. Alternatively, the subject does not consciously see the word but still processes the word subconsciously and gets the task right by guessing without remembering having seen the word. In the third case, the subject doesn't see the word and doesn't process it at all.

Conscious
Condition

Unconscious
Condition

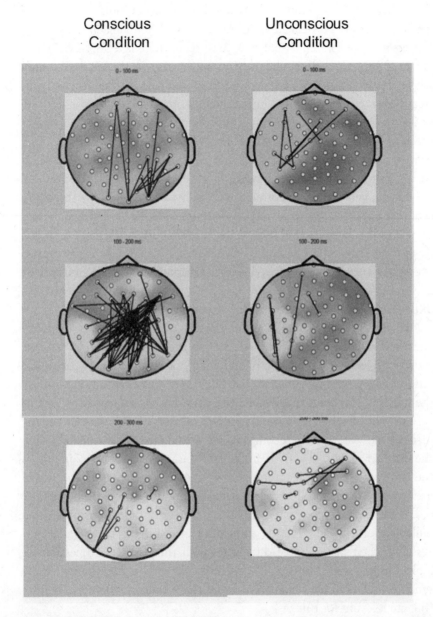

Figure 7. Differences in phase locking of oscillatory brain activity recorded from different sites of the cerebral cortex where a stimulus is consciously perceived (left panels) or just processed but not reaching the level of consciousness (right panels). The black lines connect recording sites exhibiting a significant synchronization and phase locking. Note the widely distributed network engaging in synchronous oscillations in the conscious condition.

We can measure brain activity and look for synchronization patterns between different cortical areas during the test. When subjects consciously process and are aware of what they have seen, there is a brief moment of about 200 to 300 milliseconds when remote areas in the cerebral cortex where the electrodes are located synchronize their activity in the high-frequency range that we see during meditation, as shown on the left side of this image (figure 7). The synchronization occurs very briefly and very precisely, and then it goes away again. When subjects don't consciously process what they are seeing, then there is no synchrony, or very little, as shown on the right side of the image.[41]

So it appears that one correlate of conscious perception is a transitory synchronization of neuronal responses that establishes a highly coherent pattern of oscillatory activity across the cerebral cortex. We can't say much more than that. The content of consciousness apparently is distributed over many areas, is temporarily assembled through coherence, and cannot be further reduced to a location. It is a distributed dynamic pattern. It's difficult to imagine, but that is what it seems to be.

Finally, I would like to show you possible consequences for pathology and some issues that might be relevant to therapy. In a simple task, we show a subject a pattern briefly and then make this pattern disappear. After a while, we show another pattern, or the same one again, and ask the subject, "Have you already seen this pattern, or is it a new one?" In this case the subject has to engage short-term memory to remember what the first pattern was, and then compare. Performing this task correlates with the synchronization of activity in the prefrontal region of the brain and in the parietal region—areas engaged in the management of short-term memory and attention. It requires attention and is a conscious process.

We know that schizophrenic patients who have thought disorders and hallucinations, which indicate difficulties in arranging the parallel processes in their brains, have difficulties with this task. The question we looked at was whether this also corresponds with a disturbance of the synchronized activity. One can measure the activity in the brain regions that are relevant for this task.

HH Dalai Lama: Will there also be a difference in the speed at which the synchronization takes place?

Wolf Singer: Yes. Schizophrenic patients have difficulties in producing these waves and in synchronizing them, and they also perform the task much more slowly than control subjects.

Phase Synchrony of Gamma Oscillations

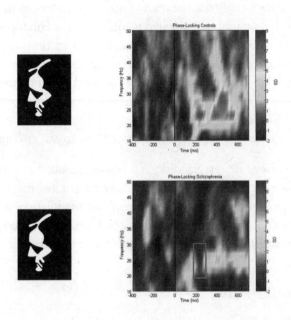

Figure 8. Comparison of phase locking of oscillatory activity between normal controls (upper panel) and schizophrenic patients (lower panel). Subjects were requested to decide whether they recognized a face in a stylized drawing (figure at left). In normal subjects, strong phase locking (light blobs in upper panel) occurs, starting 200 milliseconds after stimulus presentation, in a frequency range of 20 to 30 hertz (ordinate of the panels), a response that is lacking in schizophrenic patients (rectangle in the lower panel).

We also measured the oscillatory brain potentials and determined their synchrony during the moment when subjects see a picture for the first time and have to recognize it. In normal subjects, this produces a lot of activity in the high-frequency oscillatory gamma range, around forty hertz. But schizophrenic patients don't show this increase, and they also have difficulties in synchronizing activity in different cortical areas. This may be one of the reasons why they have difficulties in coordinating their thoughts and coherently organizing their behavior (see figure 8).

To conclude, if it is true that synchronization of these high-frequency rhythms serves to coordinate the many distributed processes in the brain, then a method of mental training like meditation that enhances synchronization should have profound effects on brain functions. Finding out what these effects are will be the goal of future research. Not all of them may be beneficial. It sometimes may not be good to synchronize things that should stay separated. But developing more synchrony might be highly effective in generating states of consciousness that differ from those we normally have when we act in a disassociated way in our environment.

Richard Davidson: Robert Sapolsky is a leading scientist who studies the impacts of stress on the brain. His pioneering studies have helped us understand the mechanisms by which stress may modulate brain function and structure and, through these influences, have pronounced effects on the body. His scientific and popular contributions are renowned throughout the world.

ROBERT SAPOLSKY *The Neurobiology of the Adaptive and Deleterious Features of Stress*

Few of us will succumb to cholera, smallpox, or scarlet fever. Instead, we die from diseases of our Westernized lifestyle, which are often compounded by stress. When the stress response is mobilized by the body because of a typical mammalian stressor (for example, a sprint to flee from a predator), it is highly adaptive. However, when activated in the modern manner of Westernized humans (that is, chronic psychosocial stress), it is pathogenic. This presentation considers this dichotomy, as well as new directions of research needed for understanding the neurobiology of stress and stress management.

During this conference a lot of experts will be talking about how to live a life in balance. Unfortunately I have no idea how to do that, but I am an expert at what happens if you don't do that: I study the effects of stress on the body. Anthropologists are always interested in what makes humans different from other animals. We now know that humans are the species that invented microwaves, ballroom dancing, and toilet training. But more than anything else, humans have invented adventitious suffering: the ability to feel pain and suffering for what once was, what will be, what could be, or what someone else experiences.

This is unique to humans, but what unfortunately is not unique to humans is what our bodies do when we feel adventitious suffering. The central concept in the study of stress is this: If you are a zebra, and a lion leaps out and rips your flesh open and you are in pain, running for your life, the things your body does then are wonderful. They are exactly what you need in order to survive. But if you are a human suffering from adventitious pain, your body does exactly the same thing, and if it does that for a long time, disease will arise.

In a sense, the reason that we, as a species, get so many diseases related to stress is that we're too smart. We can invent psychological stress. A lot of research has shown what is involved in psychological stress, including some classic animal studies done in the 1960s that I will discuss in this presentation. And by the way, I believe that the scientists who did that work thought very hard to balance the animals' pain and the good that would come of it.

In one study,[42] a laboratory rat was given a very small shock every now and then. With enough shocks, the animal developed a stomach ulcer—a disease sensitive to stress. We now know, and in fact the Nobel Prize was recently awarded for this, that stomach ulcers involve bacteria, but they depend on a stressful lifestyle in addition to the bacteria. The stress makes it difficult for the stomach to repair the beginnings of an ulcer. So the rat experienced enough stress to get an ulcer.

Another rat got the same shocks—its reality was exactly the same—but every time the second rat got a shock, it could go over to another rat on the other side of the cage and bite it. The second rat didn't get an ulcer. Thus we see that rats are close relatives of humans.

HH Dalai Lama: Is it because the rat has a chance to express the pain?

Robert Sapolsky: Exactly. What we say in my business is that it avoids getting an ulcer by giving an ulcer. A third rat got the shocks but had a bar of wood that it could chew on with its teeth. It did not get an ulcer. Again, this was a way for it to express the pain.

A fourth rat got the same shocks, but just before each shock, a light came on, warning it. Getting information about when the shock was coming, how bad it would be, and how long it would last also prevented an ulcer.

HH Dalai Lama: It prepares the rat.

Robert Sapolsky: Exactly. In the next version, a rat was trained to press a lever to avoid getting shocks; then the lever was disconnected. It didn't do anything, but the rat sat there hitting the lever and did not get an ulcer. It felt a sense of control. Finally, if the rat was in a cage with another rat that it knew and liked, and they sat together and groomed each other, it did not get an ulcer from the shocks.

These, then, are the building blocks of psychological stress. If you have no way to release your frustration, if you feel like you have no control and no way to predict what will happen, if you interpret an event as meaning that life is getting worse, and if you have no one's shoulder to cry on, this is what makes adventitious suffering stressful.

We now know how the body responds to this. To make sense of it, we need to see what the body does if you are a zebra running away from a lion. The first thing you need to do is mobilize energy. You need energy not in your fat cells for some activity next spring, but right now, going to your muscles as you run. You need to deliver that energy to your muscles as quickly as possible, so your heart beats more quickly and your blood pressure goes up. All this is based on the logic that if you can get the energy to your muscles in two seconds instead of three, you are more likely to survive.

It also makes sense that you turn off all sorts of long-term building projects in the body. This is no time to work on renovating your liver. When you are running for your life and the lion is one step behind you, it is not a good time to ovulate. During stress you stop digestion, growth, and the repair of your body. You stop reproduction, and you stop your immune system. You can do those things later if you're still alive.

All of this is wonderful for a zebra running for its life, because it is a way for its body to deal with fear and pain. But your body does the same exact thing for days and months and years because of psychological suffering. If you are always mobilizing energy, your body never gets to store it. Your muscles become weak, and you are more likely to get diabetes, which has now become a disaster globally. If your blood pressure increases while you're running away from a lion, that's a good thing. If a traffic jam causes your blood pressure to increase and that happens often enough, you will have heart disease and your blood vessels will be damaged by atherosclerosis. If your digestive system constantly shuts down, you are more at risk for an ulcer or colitis. There is a terrible, strange disease called stress dwarfism, or psychogenic dwarfism, where children are under so much psychological stress that their bodies stop growing. If you are a female mammal under lots of stress, your reproductive cycles become longer or stop all together. If you are a male, your testosterone levels go down, and you may have problems with erections. I should add that never in my life would I have thought that I'd be discussing erections here with you. But I digress . . .

If you are always under stress, your immune system is suppressed, so you are more vulnerable to infectious disease. The new field of psycho-neuroimmunology is based on the notion that your brain can affect how your body deals with disease. What we see here are two sides of a story. A normal mammal, if stressed but unable to activate an adaptive stress response, would soon die. But many diseases will emerge in a human with chronic psychological stress.

I'd like briefly to focus on the positive short-term effects of stress on the brain, and the long-term effects, which seem particularly interesting. For a short time, one or two hours, stress does wonderful things for the brain. More oxygen and glucose are delivered to the brain. The hippocampus, which is involved in memory, works better when you are stressed for a little while.[43] Your brain releases more dopamine, which plays a role in the experience of pleasure, early on during stress; it feels wonderful, and your brain works better.

Unfortunately, the opposite happens when stress has gone on for too long—for four hours, or for four years. There is less glucose delivered to your brain. Neurons in the hippocampus do not function as well. Neurons have long processes that they use to talk to other neurons, and during prolonged stress, these processes shrivel away. As we heard before, the brain makes new neurons in the hippocampus, but when there is stress, neurogenesis is inhibited. With enough stress, neurons will actually die, which is what my laboratory at Stanford studies.[44] In addition, with a lot of stress there is a decreased release of dopamine, which, as mentioned, is involved in pleasure. As a result, there is no pleasure, and that has something to do with depression.[45] Amazingly, stress makes the amygdala—a part of the brain that is involved in fear and anxiety—work better. The neurons there grow new connections and the amygdala gets bigger, and as a result, we become more trapped by fear.[46] Finally, the frontal cortex, which helps us make decisions and control our emotions, does not work well during chronic stress, and its neurons also shrivel away.[47] These are some extremely damaging things that can happen in the brain with chronic stress.

It would be easy to say, "Aha! We must have no stress in our life!" But that is nonsense. For a short period, stress does wonderful things for the brain, and we love it. It makes us feel good. We will pay money to be terrified on a roller coaster. So the question becomes, When is stress a good thing? Good stress is what we call stimulation, when there is a challenge to overcome. What is it that makes stress stimulatory?

Thupten Jinpa: We're just wondering what would be the most equivalent Tibetan term for "stress."

Alan Wallace: In other words, how do you define it? Are there two sorts, physical and mental? Or does the term cover both? We need some unpacking here, because the term "stress" doesn't translate into Tibetan.

Robert Sapolsky: Short-term stress can be physical or mental. The main thing is that it does not go on for too long and that it is not too large. It is not by chance that a roller-coaster ride is three minutes long and not three weeks long.

Psychologically, we think of stimulation as a challenge, but one where we are not helpless. We may be able to overcome this challenge. The way dopamine works is very interesting. This morning, Richie talked about how, in the United States, happiness is considered an unalienable right. I suspect that it makes more sense for our brains that we are guaranteed the *pursuit* of happiness. It turns out that dopamine is not released in the brain when you get a reward, but rather when you think you are soon going to get a reward. It is about anticipation, and thus anticipation itself becomes pleasure for the brain.

In a wonderful study, a monkey was trained to press a lever to get a reward.[48] Then conditions were changed so that when it pressed the lever, it got the reward only half of the time. After pressing the lever, while the monkey was waiting to see if it would get the reward, its dopamine reached the highest levels ever seen in the brain of a monkey. In other words, as soon as you introduce the idea of "maybe," it is so much more rewarding. When you are absolutely certain, it's boring. If there's no chance at all, you are helpless and depressed. Fifty percent is right at the point where there is challenge, but it doesn't suffocate you, and that is when we see the greatest release of dopamine in the brain.

That may seem strange. Earlier I said that a lack of control is very stressful. Here, a lack of control feels wonderful and your dopamine goes up. What's the difference? As I mentioned earlier, the research shows that if the lack of control occurs in a setting that you perceive as malevolent and threatening, lack of control is a terrible stressor. If the lack of control occurs in a setting perceived as benign and safe, lack of control feels wonderful. One of the great challenges is to understand how we can make settings that feel threatening instead become benign.

That raises a final point: Why do some of us deal with stress better than others? Why is stress for one person stimulation for another? Stress has been part of medicine for about seventy years, and it has taken about sixty-nine years to convince medicine to pay attention to it. The big challenge from now on is to understand why we differ from one person to the next, because that will teach us how to turn adventitious suffering into stimulation. Thank you for helping teach the world that lesson.

SESSION 2 DIALOGUE

In addition to HH Dalai Lama and the presenters, translators, and moderator, panelists for this session include Matthieu Ricard, Esther Sternberg, and Alan Wallace.

Richard Davidson: To begin the discussion, it would be useful to go back to a point that Wolf made. Wolf's research indicates that there's no convergence zone in the brain that is the seat of emotion, consciousness, or the self. Rather, these complex psychological functions appear to arise from the coordinated activity of many brain regions. Can you comment, Your Holiness, on the extent to which Buddhist intuitions about the mind are similar to, or different from, the intuitions that are beginning to emerge from modern neuroscience, which suggest that there is no single center for the self or for other psychological processes?

HH Dalai Lama: In some ways the understanding that is emerging in neuroscience about how cognitive functions arise seems to have similarities with the Buddhist intuition that there is no central authority, no single thing that is responsible for cognitive or mental activity. However, Buddhism does make a distinction between sensory experiences on the one hand, and mental experiences such as thoughts and emotions, on the other. Sensory experiences have a very intimate correspondence with sensory organs. For example, if you have a defective eye organ, visual experience cannot be taken over by other sensory modalities. The situation is more complex in the domain of mental experience, such as thoughts and emotion. The idea that different thoughts, related to particular content or experiences, whether cognitive or emotional, are localized in very specialized parts of the brain is contrary to the Buddhist intuition.

In Buddhist epistemology or psychology, there is no discussion of the role of the brain as such, whether in emotions or cognitive activity. Even in Vajrayana texts that mention the work of the nervous system, there is no concept of the brain having a central role in cognitive activities. It is only in the classical Tibetan medical texts that there is a recognition of the brain's primary role in human experience. Anyway, the idea that mental experience, including cognitive functions and the experience of emotions, are expressions of a much greater coordination of different regions of the brain seems to be more intuitively appealing than the idea that each specific function of the mind can be very directly correlated to a specific locality of the brain.

Wolf Singer: I find it interesting that our Western philosophies and civilizations have come to a completely different conclusion. The Cartesian view couldn't be much more different from this view. The question is, Why has this developed that way? At lunchtime we discussed this question, and it was suggested that because Western analytical science was dominated over centuries by linear models and machines, the idea arose of a brain that functions like a complex clockwork in a highly deterministic way. But we experience our brains as being creative, open toward the future, and intentional. Since linear systems that behave like clockwork have none of these properties, we are forced to postulate a "mover" to explain why brains do what they do. Because of the routine, mechanistic interpretation of the world that has dominated our way of thinking as the basis of classical physics since the Enlightenment, the Cartesian interpretation was the only way to reconcile the deterministic view with actual experience.

HH Dalai Lama: I don't know. It's difficult to say. In a way this question touches perhaps on a more philosophical and metaphysical level, which may not be that relevant to the discussion here. From the perspective of ancient Indian thought, when we think about aspects of consciousness such as cognition and emotions, the primary characteristic that comes to mind is their experiential nature, whereas in the context of neuroscience, all functions of the mind are generally seen as functions of the brain. There are two different kinds of language here. Maybe your question touches on this deeper metaphysical issue.

Part of the path of cultural influences comes from the impact of religious thinking in the past on philosophy. The notion of soul is prevalent in many cultures. Also, we all experience a sense of selfhood in day-to-day life: "I'm doing this . . . I'm doing this for myself . . . I see you," and so on. We all possess this very instinctual sense of selfhood. When we try to identify what that sense of self really refers to, we tend to assume that this is the core of our being, no matter how difficult it may be to pinpoint what it is or where it is. We feel that this is the central organizing principle, the very essence of one's existence.

In Buddhism, however, there is a lot discussion of how this mode of conceiving of oneself is unfounded. There is no such eternal, abiding principle that is truly "me," a true self. The idea that there is a soul or self, over and above the physical and mental elements that constitute our experience, is misguided. This is what Buddhism means when it talks about the negation of selfhood, or absence of selfhood. So for Buddhists, the neuroscientific explanation of how, despite all your effort, you cannot find any identifiable convergence point for self or soul within the complex network of neurons in the brain is a compelling reconfirmation of selflessness.

Wolf Singer: For us it is very disturbing.

Esther Sternberg: I wanted to follow up, Your Holiness, on your question to Robert Sapolsky about the concept of good stress and bad stress. I'd like to make that more explicit and pose the question as to whether meditation actually moves you along the stress curve. There is an inverted U-shaped curve to the stress response. When you're totally relaxed, dozing and almost asleep, you are not at peak performance. You're not performing at all. The brain centers and hormones involved in the stress response have to be activated in order to get you to the top of the U-shaped curve that represents peak performance. For example, when Wolf's PowerPoint wasn't working at the beginning of his presentation, that really made him go to peak performance because he was a little stressed. But if he was too stressed, his performance might fall off or he could freeze up completely due to overactivity of the stress response.

From everything that I've heard this morning, and after reading your most recent, very thought-provoking book, *The Universe in a Single Atom: The Convergence of Science and Spirituality*,[49] it doesn't seem that meditation puts you into that relaxed state. It seems that it increases your focused attention and moves you to the top of the U-shaped curve. Maybe what it's really doing is modulating your stress response, bringing it to an optimal point so that the nerve cells in the locus coeruleus, the part of the brain that is important for vigilance and focused attention, that gets you to peak performance, start firing optimally—not too much, not too little. I wonder if that might be part of what is happening with meditation?

HH Dalai Lama: Some forms of meditation are very difficult. One of my close friends was a very good meditator who attempted to cultivate single-pointedness of mind. He had the experience of spending a few years in a Chinese prison, and he told me that the meditation was actually harder than being a prisoner. The point is that he had to be constantly aware and attentive without losing his attention even for a moment. A constant vigilance was required.

One factor that needs to be taken into account is the intensity and quality of the meditator's motivation. In the traditional Buddhist context, meditators are highly motivated individuals who have a deep appreciation of the framework of the Buddhist path and an understanding of its causes and effects: If I do this, this will happen. They understand the nature of the path and its culmination. There is a deep recognition that the fulfillment of one's aspiration for happiness really lies in the transformation of one's undisciplined state to a more disciplined state of mind. These individuals take into account all of this context, so when they engage in meditation, they have a tremendous sense of dedication, joy, a very strong motivation, and sustained enthusiasm. But if you just tell a child, with no context at all, to start meditating, there will be no incentive, no inspiration.

Robert, you made the comment that in small doses, stress can actually raise dopamine levels, which we assume corresponds in the rat to a heightened sense of well-being or pleasure. I wonder whether there might be an analogue in meditation, specifically in the training of single-pointed attention, or samadhi, which is not uniquely Buddhist. As one trains incrementally in developing attention, a quality arises that is described as suppleness or malleability of the body and mind, and is often conjoined with a sense of well-being, perhaps even bliss. It happens very strongly when one achieves a high state of samadhi, but even incrementally along the path, there are many surges of this type of malleability together with a kind of bliss. This may be an interesting area of research, to see from the neurophysiological perspective what some of the unexpected events are that come out of such attentional training.

Matthieu Ricard: Stress usually has a negative connotation, but the positive aspect—in terms of someone who is actively trying to save his or her life—is an immediate responsiveness, a mobilization of very sharp faculties. Stress also includes the idea of inciting rumination, hopes, fears, and expectations. How to combine a heightened state of vigilance with a very serene and relaxed state of mind? It can happen because when one rests in a limpid and vivid awareness of the present moment, hopes and fears, ruminations and expectations, vanish by themselves. This is a very lucid state of mind imbued with serenity. So you can understand how focused attention, for instance, could be a very alert and responsive state without having the negative aspect of what we usually call stress.

Robert Sapolsky: That taps into a classic feature of endocrinology. People think that you secrete stress hormones when there is stress, and when there is no stress, you don't secrete them, or you secrete just a little bit. You are at baseline. It was a long-standing tradition in the field to consider baseline to be extremely boring. What's now clear instead is that baseline is a very active, focused, metaphorically muscular process of preparation for stress. The jargon used in the field is that it has permissive effects, allowing the stress response to be as optimal as possible. That's a wonderful endocrine analogue of the notion that meditation, a state of peace, is not the absence of challenge. It is not the absence of alertness and energetic expenditure. If anything, it's a focusing of alertness in preparation. It absolutely matches the endocrine picture.

Alan Wallace: I have a question for Robert. In Buddhist ethics, if you feel a desire to speak in a very injurious or abusive way, perhaps when somebody has insulted or offended you, or even to retaliate physically, you are told to restrain yourself. When the mind is clouded by mental affliction, Buddhist ethics would say, "Now is not the time to act. Let it pass and then act when the mind is more balanced." But your rats were less likely to get ulcers due to being shocked if they got relief by biting another rat, or at least gnawing on a piece of wood. I'm wondering what the implications are for human beings, when we are shocked by very disagreeable circumstances. From a neurobiological perspective, would it be good for us to go bite somebody, or at least chew on a piece of wood? Are there alternative strategies for us not to internalize the distress, get ulcers, and make ourselves mentally or physically ill? How do you see the interface between these two perspectives?

Robert Sapolsky: You are tapping into one of our most depressing features as mammals—a feature that exists across all sorts of species. The greatest way to reduce the stress response is to take it out on someone smaller and weaker. We see this not only in rats, but also in studies of nonhuman primates. Among baboons, for example, 50 percent of aggression is displacement aggression onto a third party, an innocent bystander.[50] A male who loses a fight chases a subadult male, who bites a juvenile, who chases an adult female, who slaps an infant. Almost everyone feels better afterward.

Among humans, the equivalent is that during times of economic stress, the rates of child abuse and spousal abuse increase. One of the biggest challenges in understanding ourselves as organisms that deal with problems of balance is how we can reattain balance in the least damaging, least selfish way.

Richard Davidson: Robert, do you think our capacity for regulating emotion and attention confers some potentially unique opportunities for humans as a species in ways that may be different than for other species? To a large extent, that regulation, and the brain systems that support it, really is what the mental training we've seen featured here does.

Robert Sapolsky: Yes, and I think that's the justification for all of us sitting here today: the model you presented that meditation strengthens the ability of the frontal cortex to regulate emotion.

Matthieu Ricard: One particular aspect of this is the faculty of the mind looking at itself. Instead of acting instinctively on a provocation or sensation, we can let the mind look at itself so that powerful emotions dissolve.

Robert Sapolsky: I think your use of the word "instinctive" is very important. Psychologists are very interested in moral development in children and have described all sorts of stages children can reach. It turns out that the stage individuals reach as children doesn't predict much about who will do the difficult moral act as an adult—who will actually step out of a crowd and do the right thing.

Instead, studies show that those who do this are people who were brought up in a setting where the right thing to do was emphasized over and over again during childhood: "This is what you do." "This is what you do." "This is what you do." It becomes automatic. I was not joking earlier when I talked about humans inventing toilet training. We don't sit there as thirty-year-olds and say, "What would the consequences be if I did not listen to my toilet training lessons right now?" It has become completely internalized.

When you see a news story about someone who does an extraordinary thing—the person who jumped in the river to save the child—in the interview they never talk about how they thought through what would happen if we had the sort of society where people didn't do that for each other. What they always say is, "Before I knew it, I was in the river." It had become automatic—not instinctual, but a pathway as ingrained as instinct. I think the more that becomes our imperative, the more we can overcome our limbic systems.

Wolf Singer: Coming back to the issue of meditation, we learned this morning that it is far from relaxation, with electrographic responses associated with a state of high attention. It's a strong internal activation of the brain. It is striking that this should always be associated with positive rather than negative connotations. It suggests that the brain in its default mode turns to positive states, which is surprising because we know that the brain has two systems, like yin and yang, that are responsible for positive and negative emotions. But somehow, everything I've heard so far about the contents of meditative states, along with my own personal experiences of it, is on the pleasant side. Why is that so? Why does it not happen—or does it?—that a meditative state gets you into a panic attack, for example, because you happen to activate the wrong centers in your brain? Why is it always on the positive side? And is it? Or is it not?

Matthieu Ricard: It's encouraging, in fact. When we become extremely angry and do something hurtful to others, a few hours later we say, "I wasn't myself" or "I was out of my mind." This is an intuition that although we do act in such ways, it amounts to some kind of deviation. Conversely, when you do a very disinterested and spontaneous act of loving-kindness or generosity, somehow you feel intuitively that this is more attuned to your deeper nature. In that sense, we might argue that an undisturbed state of mind would be more peaceful and positive, while hatred and jealousy are afflictive states of mind. His Holiness often says that, deep within, compassion and altruistic love are more attuned to our true nature than the afflictive emotions that emerge out of our mental constructs.

Esther Sternberg: That was in part what I was trying to address in my earlier point about the inverted U-shaped curve. But the take-home message from what I've heard about meditation up until now is not so much that it's a positive state; rather, it's a very active state, and in some cases a very difficult state to achieve. Maybe we are still thinking way too simplistically in a neurobiological sense, despite everything that you've done, Richie, and all the complex synchronization studies that you've done, Wolf.

There are other, different stress centers in the brain. Just as there are many centers that relate to consciousness and all the sensory signals that we perceive, there are many centers of the brain that relate to focused attention. There are also many centers of the brain that intrude upon your ability to have focused attention. This morning, Ajahn Amaro talked about sitting in a cross-legged position with painful knees, and the intrusive thoughts that prevent you from focusing attention. There's a part of the brain deep in the brain stem, called Barrington's nucleus, that receives inputs from the viscera that intrude on your thoughts. It sends signals to the locus coeruleus and then to the brain's stress center, the hypothalamus, because when your gut sends these signals, you need to act. You need to empty your gut, so to speak, and that takes precedence in the body's hierarchy of what it needs to pay attention to. We're always receiving signals from our organs as well as from the outside world, and there's a hierarchal competition among the signals that the brain is being asked to pay attention to. Meditation seems to be a very active process that allows you to force your brain to pay attention to something other than these intrusive signals. Maybe synchronization plays a role in getting all these different centers to talk to each other.

HH Dalai Lama: It's a very complex issue. Many of the brain's signals are very urgent, obvious, biological body signals, for example, if you need to relieve yourself or if you are hungry. Although the attentiveness of the individual may make a difference, these signals are generally very powerful.

Meditation, however, operates in what Buddhists call the mental domain. When we talk about cultivating or refining the attention, we are really talking about the mental domain. Meditation operates more at the level of adventitious or psychological suffering, rather than physical, biological pain and suffering. Generally it is very difficult for a mental activity such as meditation to completely eliminate pain at the physical level. It is possible, however, for a meditator to sometimes override physical pain as a result of deliberate or intentional mental activity. It is not necessarily the same as actually removing the pain. The pain may be there, but one could override it in such an attentive state of mind.

Esther Sternberg: That actually fits very well with the physiology. These centers deep in the brain, which receive visceral signals, are almost impossible to overcome when they're calling very loudly, but they can be suppressed by the higher brain regions when the physical situation isn't so urgent. The Buddhist philosophy works very well with what we know about how those brain stem regions are regulated by the higher brain regions, by the cortex and the conscious brain.

Richard Davidson: I'd like to take this opportunity to turn to some questions from the audience. A number of questions were addressed to very practical issues concerning how meditation can be used to influence or treat certain psychiatric disorders. One question asked us to address whether meditation practice can influence post-traumatic stress disorder to help survivors of war, torture, and great harm. I'd like to broaden that and ask whether there are particular conditions where meditation practice may not be advisable, or may be potentially harmful.

HH Dalai Lama: Given the diversity of people's mental dispositions, it's very difficult to generalize that meditation would be effective. One really has to judge on a case-by-case basis. Generally speaking, my own belief is that an individual's basic outlook on life seems to make a big difference in how he or she responds to traumatic experiences. In one of the previous Mind and Life Dialogues, there was some surprise expressed at how rarely post-traumatic symptoms were found among Tibetans who had been exposed to trauma. I often tell the story of my close friend and colleague, a monk from Namgyal Monastery who spent many years in a Chinese prison in Tibet. One day he told me that during his years in prison, he sometimes had a great sense of fear. I inquired what that fear was about. He said it was the fear of losing compassion toward the Chinese. Here is an individual who has quite a different outlook on life! It seems that this kind of outlook made a difference as to how this individual was able to withstand the imprisonment and torture.

Generally it works much better if one can prepare ahead and have some kind of preventive system in place. Once you have already experienced the trauma, it is very difficult to correct it. So I always stress the importance of proper education from early childhood. Then, when people pass through difficulties in life later, a certain kind of inner strength may prevent external difficulties from disturbing them too much. This is something we can do. This is doable.

Sometimes I encounter people, even among those I know, who tell me they have a sense of great anxiety. They seek some help from me, including blessings. But when I ask what exactly the problem is, it's a very tiny problem, not serious at all. These complaints are due, I think, to some lack of inner strength . . . And in that case I have a lot of complaints myself!

Matthieu Ricard: I once heard about a study with children from Buddhist communities in Bangladesh that are often subjected to storms and floods. The researchers found a significantly lower level of post-traumatic stress compared to children of other communities. I think it has something to do with the culture. Unlike in a very individualistic culture, where one is always worried about what could happen to oneself, this concern might be diminished when one's preoccupations are less self-centered. Consequently, one feels less vulnerable and gains confidence that one has the inner resources to deal with whatever may come one's way.

Esther Sternberg: That goes back to Robert's point about control. If you have a sense of control over the stresses that come upon you, whether that control comes from internal resources, which is best, or from external sources, perhaps that helps to protect from illnesses such as post-traumatic stress disorder.

HH Dalai Lama: That's very true.

Richard Davidson: Let me take another question from the audience that's relevant to this theme. This person asks, "Do Robert Sapolsky's comments on stress-reducing behaviors have implications for designing healthy and healing settings? Are there any Buddhist teachings on physical environment for mindfulness and compassion?"

Thupten Jinpa: His Holiness is deferring to the two Buddhists here.

Alan Wallace: There's an enormous emphasis in Buddhism on creating community. It is said that on one occasion the Buddha's attendant Ananda, being very impressed by the importance of community for one's own individual spiritual practice, said, "Lord, it seems like half the practice is sangha" (sangha being the community). And Buddha responded, "Say not so, Ananda. The sangha is the whole of the practice."

This emphasizes that we are not practicing in isolation. The emphasis on the ego, the self, the individual, which is so strong in Western society, is not an ideal in Buddhist culture. Rather, it is extremely important to cultivate environments, in terms of both human communities and a harmonious relationship with one's general environment. In that context, then, when there is a threat, whether it's invasion by a hostile force from outside or a more modest threat from a natural calamity, having a harmonious relationship with the people around you and with the general biosphere better prepares you to deal with stress without falling into post-traumatic stress disorder. You can respond with greater compassion and greater wisdom, and simply deal with reality.

Speaking very anecdotally, I was deeply impressed when I moved to Dharamsala in 1971, only twelve years after most of the Tibetans had arrived. They were still very much refugees, and yet I found the most harmonious, cheerful, and warmhearted community I'd ever encountered in my life—and not just the monks, saints, yogis, and great teachers. It was not a utopia—I don't want to be idealistic here—but I can say simply, from my own experience, that there was a sense of harmony in the community that I think must be very relevant to the rarity of post-traumatic stress disorder found there. It's partly spiritual, but I think it's also partly cultural.

Richard Davidson: So the social environment, a sangha, is preventative medicine in a sense.

Alan Wallace: Yes.

Esther Sternberg: The social environment can be either facilitated or inhibited by the built environment. I'm involved now in a project with the American Institute of Architects and the Academy of Neuroscience for Architecture, bringing architects and neuroscientists together to determine whether there are aspects of built space that either trigger the stress response or can help reduce it.

Alan Wallace: I think it's wonderful to do research in that way, but at the same time I am reminded of one of my teachers who had been a very wealthy aristocrat with multiple estates in Tibet. Of course, with the Chinese invasion he lost everything. He fled to India with his wife, and he lived in a little hut that three men built in one day for a cost of one hundred dollars. He was the principal instructor in Tibetan medicine, an extraordinarily erudite man, and I had the privilege of receiving teachings on mind training from him. He told me that in Tibet, when everything was going so well for him, he took his spiritual practice rather nonchalantly, complacently. But once he had lost everything—and quite a number of his family members had died, were murdered, or met with tragedy—he found much greater peace of mind and dedication to his spiritual practice. He exuded a sense of serenity and calm and good cheer, but his architectural environment was a hovel.

Richard Davidson: Wolf, can you foresee a time when science will produce the means to enrich meditation practice? I think it would be useful for both the scientists and the contemplatives to address this question.

Wolf Singer: It came as a great surprise to us that there were such clear electrographic correlates of particular meditative states. It told us something about what the brain can do to itself through concentration, and it probably made it more explicit to the meditators what they were actually doing. We can now tell them that they are apparently not focusing their attention on peripheral sensory modalities, as we all do, but inverting their attention to read out and engage central representations at a higher level. It would be interesting to see whether one could find a more rapid way to learn these practices using biofeedback techniques, since we now have a signature for certain meditative states, and there may be others with other signatures. It might be useful to have some external criterion that helps you find out which state you are in. I know from experience that at the beginning of the training, it's very uncertain whether one is going the right way. We know that one can generate brain states in a highly specific way if one has an indicator, a meter, that measures the coherence that one has achieved in each frequency band.

Let me give you an example that I find just amazing. Using functional magnetic resonance imaging, you arbitrarily define a point in the brain. It could be the amygdala, a piece of cortex or thalamus—it doesn't really matter. You measure the activity there, play it back to the subject, and tell the subject to try to increase this activity. Subjects lie there and try. They find out after a while that what they are doing is somehow related to what this meter does. After a couple of sessions, they become so good at it that they can deliberately increase blood flow, via neuronal activity, in specific, circumscribed regions of their brains, to the extent that they can control cursors or play Pong with somebody lying in another scanner.[51] It is amazing.

What hasn't been done yet is to ask those subjects what they are feeling when they do this. For example, if they increase activity in the amygdala, you would expect some emotions to come up or some change of internal state. I think we could learn a lot about those states and also about how the brain can control itself through the coupling of physiological parameters with self-reports.

Matthieu Ricard: I think we could learn something by examining meditation under various circumstances. As a Tibetan saying goes, "It is very easy to meditate when you are sitting in the sun with a full belly." Just the day before yesterday, we were trying the startle experiment in Paul Ekman and Robert Levenson's lab in the Psychology Department at the University of California at Berkeley. You hear the sound of a gunshot in your ears, and, normally, the instinctive reaction is to jump. We were looking for different meditation strategies that could diminish these impulsive reactions. It seemed that a state of open presence, in which your mind is vast like space and you know the explosion will be felt as a minimal incident, can allow you to not jump.

But still we tried changing the conditions, engaging in various mental states. One was being engrossed in thoughts: remembering a story of traveling somewhere and what happened on the trip. If the explosion occurs when your mind is completely engrossed in thoughts, that produces the maximum startle. In the open-presence state, when you are in the present moment very clearly and vividly and without tension, you don't need to be brought back suddenly to the present moment, so you don't jump. We're not normally exposed to such situations while remaining in a hermitage. So experimenting in such ways can, for instance, reveal to both the cognitive scientist and the meditator that being engrossed in one's mental constructs will magnify the startle response when a sudden, threatening event occurs.

Robert Sapolsky: Another way that science can help is to drag the skeptics in through the back door. I spent a lot of time with Meyer Friedman, the cardiologist who in the 1950s discovered the link between a certain hostile personality style known as type A and the threat of heart disease.[52] He was a father figure to me, always talking about his recent patients, and if someone was doing well, he would say, "I'm so happy this person has become so much nicer." He didn't say, "I'm so happy this person has a much healthier heart." One day I finally asked him, "Okay, what's the deal here? Are you in the business of preventing heart attacks or saving the world?" Instantly, he responded, "Saving the world. If it takes getting people to worry about their heart valves to be nicer to each other, I'm perfectly happy to do that." This, by the way, was a man who had his first heart attack at age fifty and saw his last patient a week before he died at age ninety-one. So he actually listened to and practiced what he preached.

Richard Davidson: Another question, which has been asked often, has to do with placebo responding and meditation. Clinical interventions are often known to exhibit a placebo effect. This question is whether there is a placebo effect in meditation.

Matthieu Ricard: In terms of meditation, placebo is like a lollipop of optimism. You eat something that contains no active substance, but you suddenly become hopeful, confident even, that it will help cure your sickness. Studies have shown that placebos have a positive effect on health. But we don't necessarily have to use such a trick. We can directly change our attitude and adopt a positive frame of mind, which has the same effect on the body without our having to swallow a blue or a yellow pill that has nothing in it. We understand that transforming one's mind is one of the best things one can do to change one's level of stress and reinforce one's immune system. It is much more sensible to achieve this through training the mind, rather than by taking a placebo.

Esther Sternberg: I agree. You said, "rehabilitate the placebo." The word "placebo" carries with it such negative connotations. It's usually accompanied by the word "just," as in "just the placebo effect." The fact is, the placebo effect is very powerful, and it's not "just" in the mind. This speaks to the point that Your Holiness made earlier, that these higher mental processes are sometimes powerful enough to suppress intrusive bodily feelings. As you said, they don't take away pain, but they can, by sending signals down through the spinal cord, actually reduce pain.

Yes, we need to think about the placebo in different terms: as a very powerful effect. I don't have the expertise to comment on whether meditation is the ultimate placebo, but I suspect that the ability to focus one's attention away from pain is a very important element of placebo.

Richard Davidson: One of the crucial issues that distinguishes placebo responding from meditation is that meditation involves an element of practice, the acquisition of a skill. You can arrange an external circumstance to elicit a placebo response, but it does not recruit the same areas of the brain that are required and are transformed when there is actual practice. From a neuroscientific perspective, I would expect that placebo responding would be far more fleeting than the effects of meditation, which would be more enduring.

Esther Sternberg: But it could be that some elements of placebo and meditation overlap. For example, the placebo effect involves learned expectations. It's conditioning. It's a more passive form of repeated learning, perhaps, than meditation, but it still involves repeated exposure to something that you expect will heal you, or, in some cases, that you expect will make you worse. There is an element of learning in a placebo, an act of thought, although we may not be aware of it.

HH Dalai Lama: Just out of curiosity, does the placebo effect extend even to more acute illness, as well?

Richard Davidson: There is controversial evidence on that. I don't think the data are clear. There are some studies that support placebo responding for certain acute illnesses. For example, there's some good evidence to suggest that an acute asthmatic reaction can be eased by a placebo.[53]

HH Dalai Lama: It is also possible that in some cases there might be individuals who are not that sick, but believe that they are very sick, and can experience a negative placebo effect.

Richard Davidson: Your Holiness, let me end on a question that one of our audience members asked: "How can we support Americans who have largely gone numb, or have become overwhelmed by constant images of violence on television, in waking up so that there can be a shift in consciousness toward a more compassionate way of being, when waking up means that they will feel pain as well as potentially the bliss that comes with compassion?"

HH Dalai Lama: Hopefully this kind of discussion can contribute toward that goal. I think usually the people who neglect positive things such as compassion are those who consider that a religious matter. Those who do not have much interest in religion or faith also neglect this value. That's why I usually try to promote awareness of the usefulness of these things through a secular approach. I think scientific findings are very powerful in this. We are not talking about God or Buddha, but simply about experimental evidence from ordinary human beings. I think that's very good.

The main purpose and the ultimate motivation of our dialogue for more than the last two decades is to help, to serve humanity through the promotion of awareness. One thing that would be really helpful is to try to bring to people's awareness the correlation that science, and medical science particularly, is finding between positive mental states and greater health and well-being. For example, you mentioned the doctor who experienced a heart attack himself, and then later helped many patients and also recognized the correlation between extreme self-centeredness and proneness to heart diseases. There is very powerfully compelling evidence coming from the science, and this needs to be shared.

Once you have a better understanding of these facts, which now have much greater scientific evidence, then your conviction in the value of these human qualities will increase and you will genuinely aspire to cultivate them. This aspiration will lead to a more joyful and happy life.

SESSION 3

CLINICAL RESEARCH 1: MEDITATION AND MENTAL HEALTH

With the advent of MBSR and then MBCT, meditative practices have shown promise in the treatment of anxiety and depression. This session, moderated by Jon Kabat-Zinn, reviews the experimental evidence for the effectiveness of MBCT in reducing relapse rates for chronic depression and discusses how mindfulness might be functioning in the brain to regulate depressive cognitions, affect, and behaviors. The different elements comprising the meditation practices and approaches are examined from the contemplative perspective, and cross-cultural issues are discussed regarding content and context and how they may serve to synergistically optimize meditation-based interventions in Western and Eastern settings.

Jon Kabat-Zinn: Good morning, Your Holiness, and welcome back. I think I speak for everybody here in saying that we are deeply moved that you have devoted so much time to our dialogues. Just being in this hall together with you, exploring the nature of mind and the potential for sanity in the human family, is an extremely rare experience. We're all immensely grateful for your guidance and leadership and for your very presence.

I hope that you're feeling somewhat better today. I know it is very stressful to be the Dalai Lama! We all admire your stamina in the service of this sometimes sorry world.

Our first dialogue of the day will be on meditation and mental health. Before we begin, I would like to offer a few opening reflections to tie this morning in with what transpired yesterday, so we keep in mind that what is unfolding in this dialogue is one seamless conversation. I believe it was Ajahn Amaro who said yesterday that what we're really getting at when we talk about residing in a deeper understanding of the nature of mind and our natural capacity for empathy and compassion is sanity, pure and simple. Allan Wallace and Matthieu Ricard both echoed this theme. Richard Davidson ended his talk with a quote from Einstein that began with the phrase, "A human being is a part of the whole, called by us 'Universe,' a part limited in time and space."[54] The quote goes on to talk about the sense of being separate as an "optical delusion of consciousness." (Editors' Note: For the full quote, see p. 55.) It might interest you to know, in terms of our theme for this session—exploring meditation and mental health— that Einstein wrote that statement not as an abstract attempt to say something about suffering, but in response to a letter he had received from a rabbi who had asked for his advice. Einstein, much like Your Holiness, was a figure of such wisdom and deep understanding that people would write to him from all over the world with their personal problems. This rabbi was asking advice on how to speak to his nineteen-year-old daughter about the death of her sister, a "sinless, beautiful sixteen-year-old child." It was in response to this inquiry about death itself and the magnitude of this kind of a loss that Einstein, with his very big mind and heart, wrote, "A human being is a part of the whole, called by us 'Universe.'" The word "whole," of course, lies at the root of the word "health," and this morning we are here to talk about mental health. The word "whole" is also at the root of the word "healing" and, as Father Thomas will recognize, the word "holy." These currents of meaning are, in some sense, all of one piece.

We spent much time yesterday visiting the human condition of suffering and will spend even more time on this topic today. We need to keep in mind how profound that suffering is and how difficult it is to liberate oneself from the second arrow of adventitious suffering, as Ajahn Amaro described it so well, let alone come to terms with the first arrow of physical pain and the actuality of untoward events. The level of suffering that clinicians and meditation teachers work with—that we all work with as part of having a body and being human—is sometimes unspeakable. The poet Naomi Shihab Nye, in her poem entitled "Kindness," speaks of the enormity of that moment when "you see the size of the cloth,"[55] in other words, when you realize the full dimensionality of the human condition, of dukkha, of the First Noble Truth. So perhaps that atmosphere will inform our conversation this morning, as we keep in mind the depth of the suffering that comes in so many different forms in a human life, and also the beauty of the calling of medicine and psychiatry and health care, the commitment to work with people who have in some sense lost confidence in their own capacity for learning, growing, healing, and transformation—and to help them to reconnect with those innate capacities and perhaps come to recognize their wholeness, in spite of all the wounds and scars.

I found that my mind this morning was cohering and decohering moment by moment with incredible rapidity over what transpired yesterday. It was as if I could watch Wolf Singer's images of all of the different parts of the brain talking to each other on different frequencies simultaneously. There were so many rich strands offered to us yesterday by all of the speakers. Thinking particularly of Wolf's description of coherence and synchronization, part of what we will hear today concerns what happens if we lose a note or two in that dynamical system that we depend on to know who we are and to feel deeply what our place might be in relationship to the world.

In Robert Sapolsky's remarkable discussion of rats experiencing stress and ulcers, we all recognized how therapeutic it might be to gnaw on a piece of wood after an insult, or at least pound a pillow, rather than biting another rat. Most species do not take their aggression to the level of murder, although some occasionally do. Our species, however, has really stretched the envelope here. The human mind can be the source of enormous suffering when it remains unexamined and attached to its own small view, caught up in greed, hatred, and ignorance. The beauty of being human is that we are not rats, or even chimpanzees. We have the potential to find hidden dimensions within our native humanity, awareness and compassion being prime among them. This morning we'll explore these dimensions for their potential value in restoring us to wholeness in the face of mental afflictions, mental diseases, and the arrows of suffering.

We are very fortunate to have as our first speaker Dr. Zindel Segal, who holds the Morgan Firestone Chair in Psychotherapy at the University of Toronto and is also head of the Cognitive Behavioural Therapy Clinic at the Centre for Addiction and Mental Health in Toronto. Zindel is a world-renowned figure in the field of cognitive therapy and the disturbance of thought processes in depression.

ZINDEL SEGAL *Mindfulness-Based Cognitive Therapy and the Prevention of Relapse in Recurrent Depression*

The advent of effective treatments for mood disorders has provided relief for many depressed patients, yet staying well and preventing relapse are enduring challenges. The clinical application of mindfulness acquaints depressed patients with the modes of mind that often characterize mood disorders while simultaneously inviting them to develop a new relationship to these modes. Thoughts come to be seen as events in the mind, independent of their content and emotional charge. They need not be disputed, fixed, or changed but can be held in a more spacious awareness. The growing empirical base for this approach suggests a 50 percent increase in relapse prevention for previously depressed patients.

I'm very happy this morning, for a number of reasons. I'm happy that my computer's working, I'm happy to be here with many of my friends, and, most of all, I'm happy for the privilege of being able to speak with Your Holiness about the sort of work that we've been doing in depression.

My talk today will focus on one specific application of our work using mindfulness and meditation to help people who have suffered with depression and prevent it from coming back into their lives. I'd like to talk about what we mean by the term "clinical depression," how it is treated, and how it has a tendency to return to peoples' lives even after they have recovered. We believe that mindfulness training can play a very important role in preventing depression from returning. I would also like to tell you about some of the research we've done to evaluate how effective this approach actually is.

The scope of the problem of depression is very large. Depression has been called the common cold of mental disorders because it is among the most frequently reported emotional disturbances that people experience, along with anxiety. The rate of depression in the United States alone is about 10 percent of the population at some point in their lives, which translates into about thirty million people.[56] The World Health Organization predicts that within five to ten years, depression will rank second only to heart disease in terms of economic and personal costs.[57] It's a very big problem with a big impact on society.

It's important to understand that we are not talking about the range of emotions that we all feel when we are sad. Clinical depression is a problem worthy of medical attention, because it really interferes with people's lives. For a diagnosis of depression, a number of different features have to show up consistently. People have to be sad every day for at least two weeks, or they have to have lost their interest and pleasure in their activities in a way that interferes with their lives. They have trouble going to work, taking care of their children, and meeting their responsibilities. Depression also interferes with sleep, with appetite, and with concentration, which is especially important when we're trying to teach people how to use mindfulness or other types of meditative practices. Thoughts of death and suicide are often a very big problem associated with depression.

Depression has a kind of trajectory or path to it. People who find themselves becoming depressed can, if they receive treatment, start to pull themselves out of the depression. If that improvement is maintained, they can recover. But even after treatment, there is still a great risk that the symptoms may return. People may be well and then fall back into a small episode of depression, or they may develop a new episode very quickly. It is almost as if it clings to them in some way. The more often they have been depressed, the more likely it is that they will suffer again.

There have been advances in the treatment of depression. The most widely used approach is to give people antidepressant medication. Medicines for depression have been effective, and they are very easy to provide to large numbers of people. But there is also psychotherapy for depression, where people talk to someone about their problems and, through that process of talking, learn ways of managing their emotions and regulating themselves to help pull themselves out of depression. Medication and psychotherapy are the mainstream approaches that are most used. Both are equally effective, which means people can help themselves in a variety of ways.

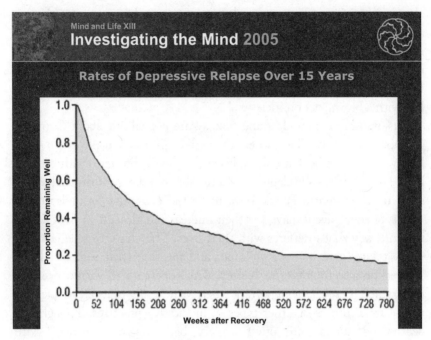

Figure 9. The risk for depression continues well beyond recovery.[58]

In a study that followed people for fifteen years, starting at a point when they were feeling well, they continued to get ill if they'd had depression.[59] So even if you've been able to stay well for five years, it doesn't mean that you're in the clear. This suggests that the effective treatment of depression involves helping people both get well and stay well. There's a paradox here: It involves persuading people who are feeling good to continue to look after themselves, yet sometimes that's not really where they want to put their energy if they feel good.

We've tried to learn how we can help prevent depression by understanding the factors that might trigger the illness to return. There are some things that we already know about what influences a relapse. The number of times that you have been depressed is a very strong predictor of whether you will become depressed again. If you're born into a family where a parent, an aunt or uncle, a sister, or a brother is depressed, chances are that if you're depressed, you will become depressed again. Significant losses are another strong trigger for depression.

These three factors are really beyond professional control. We can't do much to avoid losses or determine what family a person is born into. But there is one factor that is psychological in nature, which we can help people learn how to manage better. It has to do with cognitive reactivity to sad moods. The reactive mind of people who have been depressed seems to be very evident when they feel temporarily sad. Psychologist and philosopher William James had something to say about this problem: "Thoughts tend, then, to awaken their most recent as well as their most habitual associates . . . Excitement of peculiar tracts . . . in the brain, leave a sort of tenderness . . . behind them . . . As long as it lasts, those tracts or those modes are liable to have their activities awakened by causes which at other times might leave them in repose."[60] The idea is that once people have been depressed, even if they are feeling fine, it may not take much to tilt them back into a way of thinking that resembles depression.

One way of investigating this is to test people in the laboratory in two different mood states and look at how reactive the mind is in each. If we test people who have never been depressed, whether in a normal mood or when we make them feel sad temporarily for five or ten minutes, their level of depressive thinking doesn't really change. It may even decrease a little bit when we make them feel sad. But for people who have had an episode of depression, making them feel temporarily sad is more likely to increase depressive thinking.[61]

The extent to which people who have recovered from depression are reactive in this way when they're sad actually predicts whether depression will return over eighteen months. It's as if the sadness brings them back into a way of looking at themselves that resembles the depression.

Perhaps if we could eliminate sadness from these people's lives, they wouldn't get depressed again, but, of course, that's not possible. Instead, we try to help them work wisely with the sadness when it shows up. I'll describe some of the ways of thinking that are triggered by patients' sad moods and seem to characterize a high risk for relapse. These states of mind are automatic. The patients have very little intentional control over how they pay attention, and the moods recur very quickly. These states of mind often are avoidant or suppressive, useful in keeping things at a distance or out of awareness. There is a lot of rumination and a lot of thinking centered on the self and one's own identity. Some attitudes that characterize these states of mind are represented by statements such as "In order to be happy, I must be successful and wealthy," "Admitting to your mistakes is a sign of weakness," and "If others were to look to me for guidance, it would make me feel important."

When people are sad, these ways of thinking give them a plan for how to behave, a way to direct their energy. At the same time, they also put people at risk for a reversal in these areas, which then leaves them feeling devastated and very lost. When people reexperience sadness, they often ask themselves over and over again, "What does feeling sad say about me? Why is this sadness happening to me? How can I change this sadness?" There is a big focus on the self, and the energy used for this is taken away from other, potentially more adaptive ways of acting.

Some people see this rumination as a form of emotional wisdom, but this perception isn't accurate. Patients who were depressed in the past feel that this type of thinking has positive benefits much more than do people who have never been depressed. But when people who are in a sad mood use the strategy of rumination, they're actually less effective in solving problems that they are presented with than people who are ruminating but not feeling sad.[62]

These ways in which people who have had depression are vulnerable are some of the things we want to address in treatment. We know that cognitive therapy is effective in preventing depression. A recent study followed formerly depressed people who were well for one year to see if they relapsed.[63] One group received only a placebo pill, another group received an antidepressant drug, and another was treated with cognitive therapy. The therapy was just as effective as the medicine, and both of them were more effective than the placebo. So we know that cognitive therapy prevents relapse.

One of the ways that cognitive therapy prevents relapse is by teaching people how to identify the kinds of thoughts they have and evaluate whether they can change their degree of belief in these thoughts being true. For example, you have a thought that says, "I am a worthless person," "I am no good," or "I will never get a job." You write these thoughts down on paper, examine the situation that brought them to mind and the emotions that are present in awareness, and then evaluate the evidence. Are there some reasons why you might be able to get a job? Are there some reasons why you can't get a job? You go back and forth in this way, discussing it. This is a very traditional approach to cognitive therapy.

What my colleagues John Teasdale and Mark Williams and I have done is use the same procedures but with the understanding that cognitive therapy actually teaches patients something a little different than identification and evaluation of thoughts. In cognitive therapy, depressed patients are actually learning how to respond to their thoughts and feelings in a way that is very mindful. By writing down your thoughts you're learning how to switch out of one mode of mind into another. You're learning how to decenter from thoughts and starting to consider that they are not necessarily true and don't necessarily represent the self. You're also learning how to turn toward difficult feelings and emotions by writing them down. You have to say, "Yes, this is happening to me. I'm going to write this down." And you are working to change their degree of believability.

We believe that this teaches people a skillful means of responding to their thoughts and feelings when they are depressed. The challenge is how to do this for patients who are not currently in a depressed mood. Their depression may be gone, but they still need to learn that same emotional wisdom for dealing with judgmental or hopeless thoughts if they come to mind.

My colleagues and I developed mindfulness-based cognitive therapy, which is really an integration of cognitive therapy and the mindfulness-based stress reduction that Jon Kabat-Zinn and his colleagues developed. We've tried to put these together so that, regardless of their mood, people can still practice ways of responding to emotional experiences that involve being curious about them and moving from an automatic into an intentional mode of mind. They can have the experience directly rather than just think about it. They can learn to recognize when they might be judging their experience or trying to fix it and, through cultivating mindfulness, choose to meet the moment with non-doing and being. This is the approach that we described in our book *Mindfulness-Based Cognitive Therapy for Depression*[64] and evaluated in our clinical trials to see if there really was a clinical benefit to our theory.

The nature of mindfulness-based cognitive therapy is to help people become more aware, through systematic training in bringing their attention back to the present moment and looking at their experience from moment to moment rather than at what their minds tell them about the future or past. They start to become more aware of their bodies as places they can return their attention to and notice the changes in the flux of sensations. They explore pleasant and unpleasant events from the same perspective, and they start to work with thoughts and feelings as mental events that are not necessarily true and need not be identified with strongly.

We do this by inviting them, in the structure of a group, to practice formal meditative exercises such as the body scan; mindful stretching in yoga; and mindfulness using the breath, the body, sounds, or thoughts as the object of awareness, as well as cultivating the open focus of choiceless awareness. They continue practicing these same mindfulness meditations at home with audio recordings. We also use activities of daily living to help people become mindful in action. These activities involve developing things they can do for themselves that evoke a sense of pleasure or mastery, and also taking skillful action to prepare for relapse. We are very clear that being in our program does not guarantee that they won't get ill again, but that facing that possibility and preparing for it can limit the effects of a relapse. We also use continuous inquiry and dialogue investigating the symptoms and microexperiences of depression to help people learn to have a different relationship to these events from the one their minds may initially seize on. In informal practices, we encourage people to use all of the preceding approaches throughout their workday and leisure time so these strategies and practices become integrated into daily life. It's not a special thing they do on weekends at home for forty minutes, but something they can do every moment if they are aware enough.

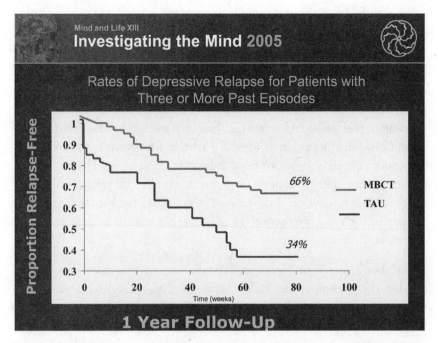

Figure 10. Training in mindfulness meditation reduces risk of depressive relapse by 50 percent.[65] TAU = treatment as usual.

We evaluated whether this treatment actually benefited these patients. In our first study we found that, among patients who were not on antidepressant medication at the time, those who participated in our program reduced their risk of relapse by 50 percent compared to those receiving treatment as usual. Of the people in the MBCT group, 66 percent stayed well, compared to 34 percent of the people receiving treatment as usual.[66]

At this beginning of the study, nobody was on medication. They could return to medication if they chose, and at the end of the study, more people receiving treatment as usual had gone back on medication than those receiving the mindfulness-based cognitive therapy. The effects were most pronounced for people who had experienced at least three previous episodes of major depression. The more recurrent the depression and the longer people had been suffering, the more benefit they had from this treatment, which is interesting.

John Teasdale and Helen Ma did another study to replicate our findings, and they had similar results. The MBCT group received greater protection from relapse: 64 percent remained relapse free after one year, compared to only 22 percent of the people in treatment as usual.[67]

In summary, our approach was designed to reduce relapse by helping patients learn how to disengage from a ruminative, reactive mind-set triggered by their sad moods. We believe that what people learn from this therapy is not to change their thoughts, but rather to change their relationship to their thoughts, as well as their relationship to their feelings and sensations. This approach is ideal for people who have recovered from depression, because they don't have to be sad to practice it. They can practice it on any mental content, because it's really the relationship that they're trying to develop. The data we've collected suggests that there's a 50 percent greater protection from relapse for people who use this approach.[68]

Jon Kabat-Zinn: Your Holiness, I'd now like to introduce our second speaker this morning, Dr. Helen Mayberg. Helen used to work at the University of Toronto, and for the past four years she has been at Emory University in Georgia. Helen is a neurologist and a neuroscientist, with a very deep interest in depression. My first encounter with Helen's work was reading about her in the *New York Times*. What she has done is so staggering that I almost fell off my chair when I read about it. We are very privileged to have Dr. Mayberg here.

HELEN MAYBERG *Paths to Recovery: Neural Substrates of Cognitive and Mindfulness-Based Interventions for the Treatment of Depression*

> *Functional neuroimaging has established that both nonpharmacological and pharmacological treatments for depression change the brain, though they change it in different ways. This presentation discusses findings from positron emission tomography and functional magnetic resonance imaging studies of functional brain changes associated with remission from depression as a result of various treatments with an emphasis on recovery facilitated by cognitive behavioral therapy. Differences between cognitive and pharmacological interventions are discussed in the context of a putative model of depression defined using*

these imaging studies. Implications of this work for understanding the impact of mindfulness meditation as an intervention in the treatment of depression are considered.

Your Holiness, I'm very pleased to be with you, and with many of my colleagues who have inspired me to understand depression as more than just a brain disease. As a neurologist, however, I'd like to tell you about depression from the point of view of the brain. That will help create a dialogue about how mindfulness, cognitive therapy, and medication affect the brain's health.

When I study the brain, I think of depression as a state of extreme imbalance between the body and the mind, and also the self. In many ways, as I've been learning with my friends here, major depression really is a manifestation of the First Noble Truth. It is an extreme form of suffering. This imbalance can be mapped to specific sites in the brain. We can use brain imaging techniques to try to understand where it lives. Here I think of the Second Noble Truth. We see that suffering has an origin; we can look to see what its cause is.

We've heard from my colleague, Zindel Segal, that different treatments for depression are available, and we can look at how different treatments work in the brain to restore balance in the mind/body system. As with the Third Noble Truth, the suffering that people experience with severe depression can end; we can identify the paths out of the suffering. We can explore where meditation might be acting in the brain to facilitate recovery from major depression and prevent relapse and, even more importantly, once balance has been restored, look at how to enhance well-being. I apologize for usurping the Four Noble Truths to talk about illness, but I do think it is a continuum.

I, too, like William James very much, for a slightly different reason. He defined depression in a way that helped me, as a neurologist, have an idea of where in the brain depression might be located. He described this intense pain of suffering as "a positive and active anguish, a sort of psychical neuralgia wholly unknown to healthy life."[69] But he said something else as well: Besides this active state of pain, in which the mind is hurting, at the same time the mind is numb. How can that be? Again it suggests that there is an imbalance in the brain. The mind hurts, but at the same time the mind is numb. How can that be, and can we study it?

111

In my laboratory, we have studied the impact of different treatments on the brain using various imaging strategies. In one set of studies we take PET scans of the brains of a number of patients who are ill and average them. Then we compare them before and after various treatments to see how the brain changes. We have done this for patients treated with medications,[70] as well as cognitive behavioral therapy[71] and, most recently, deep brain stimulation.[72]

One of the first things we wanted to understand is where suffering is located in the brain—not just the extreme of depression, but where in the brain is normal sadness? A way to approach this is by reliving a sad past experience, reexperiencing the suffering, and taking a scan during that state.[73] What happens to the brain when one feels that pain?

We see that specific areas of the brain become very active when a person is experiencing this type of mental pain. It involves a group of brain areas, the most active being the subgenual cingulate (area 25). These regions are known from other studies to be involved in the response to chronic stress and are also involved in regulating energy, sleep, appetite, libido, and various hormonal and immune reactions. Similar to the findings discussed yesterday by Robert Sapolsky, specific brain systems are activated not only in response to physical stress, but also in response to emotional stress, such as when you're feeling low.

Even as certain areas of the brain, such as cingulate 25, become highly activated, you also see deactivations or a turning down of other brain regions, particularly those responsible for active cognition. It is as if, with sadness, the emotional brain turns on, and the thinking brain temporarily turns off in a highly coordinated manner. As Wolf Singer said yesterday, it generates coherence, a coordinated response across different regions. The brain is organized to know that when something happens in one region, other regions react. When we're in a state of emotional pain, it disengages us from thinking—that is, unless we have a strategy of some kind for dealing with this kind of suffering.

I'll move now to the next step, from the healthy suffering that is part of life to the unhealthy suffering of depression. Depression is a state in which one does not have control, no matter how hard one tries. In some depressed patients, the state of depression in the brain looks exactly like the state of normal, temporary sadness in healthy people. In other patients the pattern in the brain is slightly different. This may be explained by the fact that not all depressed patients have the same symptoms. Some patients are very slow and not reactive to the environment. They cannot be engaged. In other patients the thinking part of the brain is overactive, as Zindel was telling us. I have many patients who are just in pain. They don't even have a thought to help themselves get out of the pit. We can see that the brain can be very different in different people, and those differences give us a clue as to how the brain will change when people recover.

How is it possible for the brain to display different states under the rubric of a single psychiatric diagnosis, in this case depression? The brain responds to negative challenges in the world, and when a trigger happens, the balance of the system changes. The brain doesn't just lie there and take it; it reacts. We attempt to pull ourselves out as best we can. The brain may overcorrect as it tries to think its way out of the pain. But sometimes that correction doesn't correct anything. It's just a very painful overthinking, and doesn't lead to balance. In this condition, many patients can't even begin to help themselves.

How can we assist the brain to return to and maintain a state of balance? We call it "illness," as opposed to just "suffering," because of the fact that it can't self-correct, perhaps even with training. So we try to understand where treatments act in the brain, because that may help us understand how to train the brain to reach that point through other means.

There is more than one road to recovery in the brain. I'll show you examples of two ways we can change the brain using standard treatments for depression. In the first study, in collaboration with Zindel Segal and Sidney Kennedy in Toronto, we treated very depressed patients with cognitive behavioral therapy.[74] As people recover from being extremely depressed, activity in the prefrontal cortex—the thinking brain—is turned down. This seems natural because cognitive therapy teaches patients to be less ruminative. We also see that areas of the brain that are important in excessive self-referencing are turned down. As you heard from Zindel, the idea in therapy is that it's not just about "me." It isn't just "my" pain. I can reflect it out, put it in a wider perspective, and accord less self-preoccupied attention to the sensation and to myself. Interestingly, at the same time, activity in the anterior cingulate is turned up. This is an area that is important for empathy. This raises the possibility that balance is restored by focusing less on oneself and more on others. That's not exactly what the intent of the cognitive therapy treatment is, but at the level of the brain, that appears to be the new state of balance that emerges.

With medication, on the other hand, it is a very different story. Medication can work on the same brain areas, but it changes them in a different way. It restores balance using a different strategy. Activity in certain areas of the brain is turned down, particularly in the subgenual cingulate (area 25), the area associated with intense sadness in our previous study. One interpretation is that turning down the subgenual cingulate activates the frontal cortex and releases the thinking mind. Interestingly, in contrast to cognitive therapy, which seems to uniquely target the medial frontal cortex and the anterior cingulate (areas of the brain that are important for self-awareness, insight, and attention to others, and thus less self-preoccupation), medication uniquely influences regions mediating the stress response and the state of the body (the brain stem, basal ganglia, hippocampus, and subgenual cingulate).[75] Activity decreases in these brain areas, which we think regulate the body state of suffering, and in turn, the mind is restored to balance. This reinforces what I said earlier. When one is suffering in a normal, healthy way, activity in the body components of the brain increases, and the thinking brain—the cortex—is turned down. With medication, the exact inverse happens as you recover. The body states turn down and the cortex is freed; the numbness is gone.

This balance, moving in one direction or the other, shows how these regions are highly connected. Whether we study it in this very simple way or through the very elaborate dance of different brain regions interacting with one another that Wolf Singer was describing, we've identified the brain areas that provide the substrate for the interlocking of emotion and thinking.

We also have some very depressed patients who do not respond to talk therapy, medication, or shock therapy. They have tried every available treatment. One patient describes his state of perpetual illness as "a gnawing agony in the pit of your stomach; a painful self-loathing that consumes all your energy, making it impossible to pay attention to anything else." It is a mental pain, but for him it seems to live in his stomach, to the point that he actually holds his stomach. At the same time, his mind is a blank. This is very interesting. Medically speaking, there is no problem with his stomach or with his heart. But for many patients, depression becomes an enslavement of the body, to the point where the mind has no clarity at all. All they have is pain, and the rest is totally blank.

We have a group of these very sick patients, and we've done something quite radical with them. We believe that the source of the problem lies in the subgenual cingulate, the area of the brain that becomes active when even healthy people become sad. It's as if it becomes stuck. So we make a small hole in the skull and insert a very small wire down to this spot in the brain, one on each side, while the patient is awake in the operating room, in order to try to turn off the pain. We attach the wires to a battery pack and stimulate, or at least interrupt activity in, this area of the brain. The idea is to interrupt the electrical circuit that is producing this sustained negative feedback.[76] When we did this with the patient described above, he said that the pain suddenly seemed to leave. This was very surprising and extremely dramatic. But more important to the hypothesis of the experiment, as his sense of the pain drifted away, his thinking suddenly came back to life and he became more interested in what was happening in the operating room. He'd been in the operating room for three hours with us, but only with the acute stimulation did he become aware that there were things for him to pay attention to. The enslavement of the mind by the body, caused by different parts of the brain fighting with each other, had been changed. Another patient, who was recovering after having been treated with the stimulation over a period of two months, told us, "The most fundamental change that I can see is that it isn't like something has been added. No, something has been taken away. That heavy, sinking vortex feeling was always there in some form or another. And now it is gone."

But it is not a return of total health; as the second patient described it very clearly, "It is as if instead of being in a very deep canyon, you are now up on a ledge. You look around, and you know it is still eight hundred feet to where you want to be, but you are not in a hole anymore. Now it comes down to you." He is saying that now it is possible for him to participate, something isn't fighting him anymore, and now he can work to achieve better health.

We know from both imaging studies and other neuroscience experiments that the interactions between these brain regions are not coincidental. We know how they are anatomically connected, and we can see that the way different regions change, like a dance to restore balance, involves some very specific groupings. It would seem that brain regions that control the state of the body must be balanced with regions that control thinking and how we relate to others, to the world, or to our senses. But very importantly, it's not just about body and mind, but about how they are brought into self-awareness and insight. Different treatments work on different combinations of these regions.

I want to point out that, despite the fact that we draw many of our inferences from studies performed in animals, rats are not people. While they have many of the same drives and body responses, rats are wired differently from people, particularly in terms of self-awareness and insight. Rats actually do not have brain regions equivalent to those we believe allow people to understand themselves and their relationship to the outside world and other people. Rats have a frontal lobe, but they do not have all of the same parts or the same connections. This is an opportunity to understand what makes us human; for instance, what gives us the capacity for compassion as part of the road to healing. It also helps us know the limitations of what we can and can't do with rats. They serve a very useful purpose for understanding many things, but not all things.

I close by coming back to thinking about where mindfulness fits in. Every day we are confronted with many challenges. Zindel discussed common triggers that can cause depression to return. However, we also experience challenges that may trigger suffering but don't necessarily put us on the path to illness. In both cases, the brain may still adopt these imbalanced states. It's how we're constructed. Mindfulness and other forms of meditation may be helpful for not allowing an imbalance of this kind to go too far. They might help limit the imbalance, allowing us to feel suffering while also tempering it. At the same time, mindfulness and other forms of meditation may also facilitate restoring balance.

More importantly, beyond even restoring balance, which is what we focus on as doctors, the real goal whenever possible is to enhance well-being beyond the normal. As physicians, we're happy when we simply get patients back on an even keel; unfortunately, many times we don't even get that far. We have to settle for less than optimal outcomes because that is the best we can do. For someone with cancer, we may have to settle for getting them a few more years, rather than expecting a cure. For many mental illnesses and neurological illnesses, enhancing the patient's quality of life is enough, and the limit of what we can provide. But in fact, our goal is always more than that. In the case of depression, our goal is recovery from the depressed state, but then, once the patient is better, hopefully he or she will continue to grow beyond what we might call "normal." Hopefully our treatments will be able to catalyze a robust well-being, which in turn will allow the imbalances to be less profound when suffering does show its face.

SESSION 3 DIALOGUE

In addition to HH Dalai Lama and the presenters, translators, and moderator, panelists for this session include Jan Chozen Bays, Jack Kornfield, and John Teasdale.

Jon Kabat-Zinn: We have just heard an extraordinary account of the evidence that it is possible in some cases to relieve a kind of suffering that was thought to be completely impossible to influence. We are beginning to understand deeper and deeper levels of the brain's functioning and what particular areas actually do under various conditions of disease and affliction. Your Holiness, does what you've heard bring out any intuition on your part about the potential of contemplative practice to bring us, as Helen was suggesting, not just back to baseline but to higher states of well-being?

HH Dalai Lama: Strictly speaking, Buddhist practices are really aimed at the attainment of what Buddhism calls liberation. Buddhist contemplative practices may have an effect in the health domain because much of our suffering, particularly psychological and emotional suffering, results from what is understood to be a distorted way of relating to the world, a distorted way of seeing and being. Many of the practices are really aimed at overcoming or dispelling this form of distortion and delusion. The process of practicing Buddhism, of aspiring for liberation by engaging in the practices, may also involve the restoration of health as a by-product. But as to the details of how the practices affect health, I have no idea.

Jon Kabat-Zinn: Let's begin the dialogue this morning by inviting comments from Dr. John Teasdale, from Cambridge University in the United Kingdom. John is one of the world's experts in cognitive modeling of rumination, depression, and affective disorders, and a co-developer, with Zindel Segal and Mark Williams, of mindfulness-based cognitive therapy. John is also in training to become a meditation teacher in the vipassana tradition in Theravada Buddhism, so he stands in two worlds in a truly remarkable way.

John Teasdale: Your Holiness, I'd like to consider the issue of treatment dissemination: how we can deliver mindfulness-based cognitive therapy effectively to the many people who might benefit from it. The clinical trials we've conducted show that this treatment can be very helpful to people,[77] but in delivering it to the potentially millions of people who might benefit, there is a real issue about how we preserve the effectiveness of the treatment and its integrity. The way we respond to this challenge will very much reflect our understanding of what is going on in mindfulness-based cognitive therapy to achieve the benefits it demonstrates. I'd like to consider two broadly different views of what is happening.

One view is essentially that we are training people in techniques. We are giving them a set of skills to regulate their attention: how to focus it in a particular way, sustain that focus, and then potentially disengage from unhelpful topics such as ruminative thinking and refocus attention on more neutral topics like the breath or body sensations. If we take that view, that it's a skills training technique, there may not be too many difficulties in spreading this approach. It's a relatively straightforward task, and we can make use of recordings of guided meditations and other supports that are available.

However, there is another broadly distinguishable view: that, beyond the benefits of skills training, patients make important changes in their understanding of the nature of their suffering. They shift their view of unpleasant and painful experiences, and this change in view leads to a change in how they relate to those experiences. They learn to relate to emotional pain and sadness in ways that will not get them so stuck in the adventitious suffering that we have talked about. From this perspective, the role of meditation in the program is more than simply training attention regulation skills. It's a way of embodying and exploring this different view and this new way of relating.

This more sophisticated view has more complex implications for the dissemination of treatment. It is also more subtle and may require more skills and understanding on the part of instructors, particularly because a lot of the shifts that we're talking about occur at an implicit level and are affected by the instructor's whole way of being.

Regardless of our individual opinions as to whether the simpler or the more subtle view of the way MBCT works is more accurate, opinions and thoughts aren't facts, as we tell our patients. If we really take seriously the issue of disseminating these treatments widely, we need more empirically based evidence as to which of these views is the most appropriate.

Looking to the cognitive behavioral tradition from which mindfulness-based cognitive therapy is drawn, there are a number of strategies we could use to determine what the effective mechanisms are in a treatment. These strategies could help us decide between these two alternatives. If we can be more explicit about the key change mechanisms, it may also help us enable instructors to be even more skillful, so that we move from the intuitive and the implicit to the explicit and the well described.

Cognitive behavioral therapists have adopted three broad strategies of research to investigate treatment mechanisms. The first is to identify the actual processes that mediate change and the variables that carry the effects of change. In the case of mindfulness-based cognitive therapy, we might look at the brain changes that seem to predict and carry the effects, as Helen described so elegantly. At the psychological level, we already have some evidence that mindfulness-based cognitive therapy works through its effects in increasing mindfulness and self-compassion.[78]

A second strategy is called disassembly, or component analysis. Essentially, we begin to take the whole package apart. We might, for example, take just the skills training component of mindfulness-based cognitive therapy, strip down the complex package to just the techniques in attention regulation, and see whether we still get the same effects.

The third strategy is potentially the most radical. We try to identify the effective ingredients in this complex package, much of which comes from traditional meditation procedures. But we start again and build up from the bottom, assuming that the traditional procedures, which have evolved over millennia for one purpose, may not be the most appropriate vehicle for delivering what we need now. It is not quite reinventing the wheel, but perhaps reinventing the pneumatic tire, so that we have more efficient, more focused, and more effective ways of achieving the ends we want. It is as if to say, yes, we've benefited enormously from the traditions, but perhaps the role of this generation is to change things, to introduce some new technologies here.

HH Dalai Lama: I wonder whether it is really necessary to choose one model as opposed to the other. The strategy of mindfulness-based cognitive therapy could be seen differently in the context of different patients. For some individuals, the problem is much deeper. If an individual's basic orientation, the way he or she understands life and relates to others, is dysfunctional, then a method is required that will change that basic way of relating to the world. For others, the problem arises more as a result of rumination—habitual uncontrolled thought processes. Here, the approach could be more technique oriented, where you simply teach the person a skill to disengage.

John Teasdale: I think your point is absolutely spot-on. Within the cognitive behavioral tradition, the question that's usually posed is, What intervention will be effective for what person, in what context? We recognize that different people may have different needs; but if we could identify the kind of people for whom one approach is most appropriate and attune the techniques to them, that may offer the greatest effectiveness. The other possibility is to use a stepped care approach. We would start by teaching everybody techniques, and those who can benefit, do. We then add the more subtle changes in understanding and relationship for those who require something further.

HH Dalai Lama: The challenge with the second, more complex model is the need for a sensitivity to what kind of content you need to provide, because you are trying to change someone's basic outlook on life. For example, if one of the big problems underlying an individual's state of mind is a very strong grasping at, or identification with, some form of permanence, then what's needed is a deeper recognition of how mental events are transient. They come and go. That can be seen as a universal truth, which has no religious dimension, and it can be helpful.

Alternatively, if an individual's grasping is primarily focused on a very strong sense of self, then the Buddhist teaching on no-self could be very beneficial. But if you bring in Buddhist teachings in a context where the person has no Buddhist leanings, it raises sensitive questions of religion and spirituality.

Your third strategy raises a crucial question about whether the traditional teachings on meditation practices need to be adapted in today's context. Insofar as the primary purpose of the traditional Buddhist meditation practices is to overcome afflictions of the mind and deal with destructive emotions such as anger and hostility, these two-thousand-year-old practices do not require any modification because the problem remains the same, and the solution or therapy remains the same. However, that is not the context of our discussion here. What we are trying to do here is identify aspects of the traditional meditative practices that can be adopted in the domain of health. And here, new scientific research in cognitive behavior therapy is really worthwhile for seeing which elements of this practice can be more effectively adapted to the specific purpose of health.

Jon Kabat-Zinn: This might be a perfect time to expand the conversation to our other panelists. We've made a point of asking Western dharma teachers in the different Buddhist traditions to be part of this panel, including two wonderful teachers who many people know: Jan Chozen Bays and Jack Kornfield.

Jan Chozen Bays is both a Zen teacher and a pediatrician. She also works with people with post-traumatic stress from childhood abuse of various kinds, so she is very familiar with the domain of suffering expressed in depression. The Western dharma teachers also function, in a way, as therapists. As Ajahn Amaro said yesterday, the Buddha is spoken of as the doctor of the world. Jan, I think it might be very interesting to talk about what you experience in your teaching in light of John Teasdale's questions. You must see many people with mental health problems since you work with the general population. Do you see your approach to meditation practice being adequate in this context, or do you feel that it needs to be modified in some sense in order to speak deeply to the heart of each human being?

Jan Chozen Bays: I find that many people come to Zen practice who are depressed, and that they use long meditation retreats as a way of self-medicating. By the end of the retreat they feel much better, but when they go home they relapse back into depression. As a physician, if I see that people seem to be depressed, I often recommend that they try medication. They may feel self-critical about trying medication, but I explain that it's like diabetes. If your pancreas runs out of insulin, it's not your fault. If your brain has a difficulty in its electrical circuits or its chemistry, it's not your fault. Sometimes if those people take medication, they then have enough energy to meditate. They regain some hope and some mental clarity. So the temporary relief of suffering through medication can inspire them to begin to undertake the path to liberation. This combined approach of medicine and meditation can be very good.

Depression is not a new problem. In the Pali canon, Mara talks to the Buddha in the voice of what we call the inner critic. When the Buddha is lying down relaxing after a long day of meditation, Mara comes and says, "You're being so lazy! Why aren't you working harder for liberation?" And the Buddha says, "Well, I'm lying down and meditating." And then the opposite occurs: When the Buddha is working very hard at his meditation, Mara comes to him and says, "You're working too hard! You should relax. You should enjoy your life as it is." These critical, disparaging, and despairing voices inside a human being are very old, and the Buddha experienced them too.

In Buddhism this inner critic is called skeptical doubt, and it can destroy a person's spiritual practice. Each religious tradition has a different form of the inner critic. The Catholic inner critic says, "You could be sinning and not even know it!" The Protestant inner critic says, "You're not working hard enough. Work harder!" until that becomes a problem. The Jewish inner critic says, "Your mother is not happy! You're doing something wrong." People ask me what the Buddhist inner critic says. I think the Buddhist inner critic says, "Well, that was not an enlightened thought! That wasn't a compassionate way to be."

It's very helpful to get some perspective on these self-critical energies. I see depression as being stuck in the First Noble Truth. People are stuck in suffering and can't move on to the good news that there's relief from suffering. The Buddha defined hell as physical and mental suffering with no hope of relief. When hope is lost, then people are in hell. Treatments such as medication, electrical stimulation, or mindfulness-based cognitive therapy give people some hope so they can move on to the Second, Third and Fourth Noble Truths.

I also find that each aspect of the mind has a core of truth in it, even if it has become neurotic and makes us ill. There is a curious research finding that people who are depressed are more accurate in predicting games of chance. Isn't that interesting? If you're pessimistic, you're more realistic, at least about games of chance . . . like life. If we could take the kernel of truth from depression and purify it, it would be that there *is* human suffering, and we need to be realistic about it and face it with a certain patience. People who are depressed often have a patient endurance. If those two qualities of realism and patience can be refined, they can be very helpful in meditation practice and in daily living.

I'm also very concerned about the media, because I think that our human organism was designed to take in only so much suffering. For tens of thousands of years we lived in small tribes or villages that had maybe one or two hundred people. But now, through the media, we're bombarded with much broader human suffering. To cope with that and live a life of freedom and happiness, we need extraordinary help, extraordinary medicine. I feel that the Buddhadharma offers that kind of extraordinary help and is very necessary at this time.

Jon Kabat-Zinn: Perhaps we should hear from Jack Kornfield, a very beloved and widely respected meditation teacher in the Theravadan tradition. We're delighted to have you lend your voice and wisdom to this dialogue, Jack. You have a huge amount of experience with people who come to the dharma for one reason or another, and with this whole area of what is, in fact, true mental health. What is the path to it, and what are the obstacles to it, in your experience?

Jack Kornfield: I've worked and trained as a clinical psychologist and also as a meditation and dharma teacher. I hope to contribute to our conversation particularly from the contemplative perspective. Of course, these fields cannot be separated. Many of the people who seek dharma training and contemplative instruction also deal with the need for healing of trauma, depression, anxiety, or fear, and these problems come to light as a natural part of their meditation training.

There's a growing sophistication in the neurosciences. We do not simply speak of the brain; now we can study the relationships of many structures, areas, and dimensions of the brain and its activity. In parallel to that, what we need in this conversation is a growing sophistication relative to meditation. I want to underscore that there is no such thing as "meditation." There are many distinct meditative mental trainings. That's a better phrase, because there is no single meditative state. There are dozens of trainings of mindfulness—mindfulness of body; of physical elements;

of senses; of feelings, thoughts, identity, and relationships—and trainings of directed and undirected mindfulness. There are hundreds of forms of concentration practices: visualizations, mantras, development of positive emotions, contemplations, and so forth. For our science to develop, it has to become very clear which particular mental training we're studying, and whether we are studying the states it produces or the long-term traits.

In Buddhist psychology, mental health is simply defined as a decrease of unhealthy states of mind and an increase of healthy states of mind. The Abhidharma elucidates fifty-two mental states. Some are unhealthy qualities, including hatred, grasping, jealousy, confusion, rigidity, addiction, and worry. On the other side are qualities that define human health, among which mindfulness is key and which include flexibility, clarity, love, fearlessness, and ease. The Buddhist psychological training, or treatment, if you will, shifts us from what is suboptimal—the entanglement in confusion, addiction, rigidity, and so forth—toward what is normal, with a greater increase of healthy states and, finally, to extraordinary mental health, well-being, and inner freedom. What we need to do is to study the specific ways of training for each of these different capacities, and how human beings can help one another to train in them.

In addition to inner training, another of the principles of Buddhist psychology is the use of collective practices that are communicated from one being to another in a supportive web of relationship. My friend, the writer Anne Lamott, once said to me, "My mind is like a bad neighborhood. I try not to go there alone." Mental health is not possible in isolation. Connection with sangha, or community, and the collective aspects of human transformation is part of what makes mental health possible and sustainable.

Now let us talk about identification. Zindel spoke about releasing strong identification with negative thoughts and feelings. In Buddhist psychology there are two kinds of identification. One is taking an experience as self: "my thoughts," "my car," "my country." The other, as the Abhidharma notes, is a comparative social identification: "I am better than or worse than . . ." The creation of identity is mysterious, and also central to the understanding of human freedom. As scientists, it will be important for us to study the ways we can shift identification. There is an extensive series of practices in Buddhist psychology that work to release identification from the body, from emotions, from pain, and from social conditioning. In developing this new field of contemplative neuroscience, it will be revolutionary to study identification: how we construct and can change, shift, and release identification with the sense of self.

In using Buddhist psychology for healing, there are four major dimensions to attend to, which follow the four foundations of mindfulness. The first is mindfulness of the body. Trauma, depression, and anxiety are held in, and revealed through attention to, the body. When people describe their depression or a trauma, I might ask, "How do you experience that in your body?" Their bodily attention can begin to release memories and emotions in a mindful way that brings transformation and relief. Then, sometimes the healing attention needs to focus on the second foundation of mindfulness: pleasant, unpleasant, and neutral feelings. What are these feelings? How are they experienced inwardly? How are people working with vulnerability, grief, anger, or fear, and how can that be shifted? Sometimes the focus is on the third foundation of mindfulness: the mental thought process, cognitive discourse, and one's relationship to the story-telling mind, whether contraction, identification, belief, or release. The fourth foundation is mindfulness of the dharma, which focuses attention on the laws and principles of experience. With this level of mindfulness we see the processes of conditioning, of impersonality, impermanence, and emptiness. We gain perspective. As we continue to scientifically study mindfulness, we need to acknowledge which of these different dimensions we're working with. We have to recognize that healing and transformation don't work fully if one of these dimensions is left out. If you attend only to body, or only to cognitive thinking, without including the other foundations, then you don't really come to integration or liberation.

In Buddhist understanding, another central principle is an emphasis on the quality of intention or motivation as a key to the future results of our experience. Motivation can become very subtle. In Buddhist psychology, intention is described in milliseconds and even in microseconds. Well-trained attention can separately track intention and sense its relation to the parallel mental processes of sense perception, recognition, memory, cognition, and response. There are intriguing ways we could begin to study how intention works. I would like to see a study, for example, of the neurobiology of the same act done with different intentions, or a study of brain changes as we train and transform our intentions.

Wolf talked about brain oscillation and synchronization. There is a parallel inner practice that could help us understand this dimension. In certain monasteries there is an intensive meditative training that shows us how to experience our world as vibrations. When attention to this level becomes highly developed and the mind concentrated, sound is experienced as a series of vibrations at the ear and then at the heart. Then sight and thought can be experienced as vibrations. You can even sense yourself about to think. It's like a little burp that wants to come, a prethought vibration that signals that a thought is about to emerge from the unconscious or the mind. It would be interesting to study subjects who've learned how to deliberately synchronize their inner vibrations or in some way work with the vibratory aspect of consciousness.

When we speak of compassion or love for one another, we tend to lump these states all together. But there are many forms of compassion—loving-kindness, joy, gratitude, forgiveness, and equanimity—and each has different depths and different trainings. I would like to see a study that differentiates them. What happens when you teach a joy meditation to people who are depressed, as opposed to when you teach them a meditation on friendliness or a mental practice of gratitude? We could take these different contemplative practices and see which are most effective in different circumstances.

Father Keating spoke about silence. In the Buddhist tradition, one of my teachers described twenty-one levels of silence, including silence of darkness, luminous silence where the body or space becomes filled with light, and silence with and without content. Again, these may be associated with brain states and traits that we can investigate, differentiate, and learn from. Most importantly, they point to vast inner possibilities. Western psychology has been so focused on pathology and the healing of disease that we have neglected our human potential. I would love to see research that goes further, that investigates the extremes of mental well-being and, ultimately, the nature of consciousness itself. There is much to learn about consciousness from contemplative practice. In meditation we can turn and shift identity from the content of experience to consciousness itself. We can examine consciousness and learn how to release identity from consciousness, and come to a kind of freedom beyond any states.

From the work of Zindel, Jon, Richie, and others, we can already see great fruits from the initial years of studies bridging neuroscience and

Buddhist contemplative knowledge. I believe that studying these other dimensions of the contemplative tradition will open powerful new understandings of mind and mental health.

Alan Wallace: I had the very great privilege of working for years with His Holiness's personal physician, Dr. Yeshe Dhonden. Generally speaking, in the Tibetan context, and I think this was also true in classical India, when people had physical problems or mental illnesses their treatment was primarily in the hands of the physician. Herbal compounds were given for depression and for various types of mental imbalances. On many occasions during the thousands of hours that I translated for Dr. Yeshe Dhonden, he would tell people who came in with strong psychological problems not to meditate, because the meditation might exacerbate the problems they were experiencing.

Generally, in the traditional context, when a patient is psychologically below normal, a physician would draw on traditional Tibetan medicine, or ayurvedic medicine in classical India, to heal pretty much everything we've been discussing in this conference. I totally agree with His Holiness that it's appropriate to adapt mindfulness-based therapies in ways that have never been used before, and to do that we need ingenuity, creativity, and fresh thinking.

But I want to cordon off that area of creativity and further research and go back to your comment, Helen, when you described parts of the brain correlated with depression as the substrate of the Second Noble Truth. I would be astonished if any form of suffering that anybody has experienced had no neurophysiological correlate, no immediately preceding physical event that triggered the actual experience of suffering. In the Buddhist worldview, there will always be a biological cause that gives rise to human suffering, human joys, and so forth. But it would be misleading to identify that as the Second Noble Truth—the source of suffering. There are points where that's very valid; for example, in cases of brain injury or severe chemical imbalance. In such cases it's very likely that altering one's worldview, shifting one's attitudes, or practicing meditation will be of no avail. Sometimes the physiological determinant will override anything that talk therapy or meditation can do, in which case the physiology is the most important cause of that particular suffering in that clinical setting.

For myriad other forms of depression or mental imbalance, the primary cause is not brain damage. I imagine there are probably hundreds of thousands of people in Pakistan right now who are very depressed. They've gone through a tremendous tragedy. For any of them, you could do a brain scan, and Wolf could locate the synchronicity, and you could find the particular parts of the brain responsible. But to say they are suffering because of their brains is not a meaningful answer. Even though a cause is there, the treatment is to bring them some food, help them rebuild their buildings, care about the loss of their loved ones, and so forth. That's one case where the most important cause of the depression is not neural patterns, but environmental factors.

In some cases, it may be one's attitude, self-concept, or worldview that is triggering the brain mechanisms. It may be the way one was brought up or the neighborhood where one is living. Coming back to our beloved William James, who is one of my heroes, during the 1860s when he was receiving his medical training at Harvard—he become a medical doctor before he did all the other great things in his life, despite his medical training—he was indoctrinated to believe that the brain is solely responsible for everything that happens to the mind, and that the mind has no top-down influence on the brain. He felt absolutely disempowered by this. He said he felt as if he was not an agent—that he was acted upon but not an actor. He fell into a deep and enduring depression in which he was virtually catatonic, catalyzed by this worldview that reduced his whole identity to brain function, at a time when they knew virtually nothing about brain function. So when he talks about depression, he is talking about his own experience. The only way he extricated himself from that deep depression was by shifting his worldview. In 1870, at twenty-eight, he recorded in his journal that, after reading an essay by the French philosopher Charles Renouvier, he had come to believe that free will was no illusion and that he could use his will to alter his mental state. He need not be a slave to a presumed biological destiny, as he had been led to believe during his medical education. "My first act of free will," he wrote, "shall be to believe in free will." From that time on, he took active steps to combat his affliction by psychological means.[79]

Helen Mayberg: Let me correct something from my presentation. One of the dangers of being a novice student of Buddhism is that you are a novice student. My feeble attempt to link depression and treatment with the Four Noble Truths was probably a bad idea. My use of metaphor usually gets me in trouble, and I think this is an example.

What you are saying is fundamentally true. We could get into this philosophically: How do we know what we know? What is cause, and what is effect? What is chicken, and what is egg? Is mind outside of brain? However, I don't think I'm a good person to engage in that discussion. As a neurologist, I'm fairly concrete. You have to be concrete to sign up as a neurologist. I was trying to illustrate that there is a neurological correlation with a mental state, not a cause. That was my mistake in referring to it incorrectly as the Second Noble Truth, which is the origin of suffering. There is an imprint at the brain that gives us a signal.

"Depression" is a problematic word. We all believe we know what it means because we toss it off so easily: "Oh, I'm depressed; I got a run in my stocking." At the same time, when we are describing severe psychopathology, we presume that because the word is descriptive, it offers a definition as well. We move to the next step and presume that because we can take a picture of the brain and "see" depression, it therefore is real.

It has been occurring to me more and more, not just from these conversations, but also from my work, that when the brain is in clearly different states—and the *Diagnostic and Statistical Manual of Mental Disorders*[80] says they are the same pathology—maybe our definition of the psychopathology is too broad. We need to redefine the nature of suffering to understand how it may be a condition more like dukkha, instead of a disease with a physiological cause as specific as something like a brain lesion.

That is not to deny that true psychopathology exists, or that the patients I take care of do not suffer from a brain disease. I believe very strongly that they do. But I also see patients who, with focused attention and by acquiring new skill sets, can bring themselves out of it in the same way that William James did when he decided to focus his attention from inside to outside. The ability to focus attention means your brain is in a different state. Maybe we ought to understand those as different definitions of illness. What I've learned from all of you is that maybe we have to start making those distinctions more strongly. That will allow us to focus attention on how to handle ourselves in a world with natural levels of suffering, and help us not stigmatize people who don't have the brain capacity to even start. Those are two separate items.

Jon Kabat-Zinn: Here's a question from the audience directed at you, Helen: "Does the heterogeneity in brain systems underlying a 'single disease entity' such as depression, seen on functional imaging, help predict different targets for deep brain stimulation versus cognitive therapy or drug therapy?"

Helen Mayberg: I hope the person who posed that question will be the reviewer of the grant I sent in again last week! I think we waste a lot of time in clinical medicine fighting with each other to insist that our own theories are the strongest. Once we determined that the heterogeneity in the brain scans was real, not somebody being stupid and not knowing how to analyze their data, it put us in a position to ask a very different question. Heterogeneity exists. That means our definitions of clinical depression must not be adequate, or at least not specific enough. One can then ask of the data whether the variations the brain scans actually predict which people will best respond to different treatments. The answer is that it looks like it does.[81]

So we look at a state of the brain in response to a trigger, and in my personal work, this area, cingulate 25, becomes the nexus of the problem. How the rest of the brain responds to a trigger, as a function of your early life experience, your genes, and your temperament, indicates that what the brain is showing us is not the illness, but what the brain is trying to do to restore balance. We can enhance that through different teachings or different kinds of treatment.

Consider the metaphor of heart disease. We all know that you shouldn't smoke and that high cholesterol is a bad risk factor. You should exercise; you shouldn't eat too many cheeseburgers. But at the point when you have the heart attack, it's really easy to make the diagnosis that your heart muscle has died. At that point, you are no longer dealing with probabilities. Instead, a specialized test is done to determine the nature of your problem and to match it to the appropriate treatment. For example, if you have one heart vessel clogged, you need to have that single heart vessel opened. Somebody else, who has five heart vessels blocked, will need a different kind of treatment. The heart itself is telling us how it should be treated. Of course, you would like to promise to exercise more and eat fewer cheeseburgers—but only after you survive and have had whatever surgery you need. In cardiology, there is no problem with doing a test to identify how to optimize the short-term and longer-term return to health. We have to take the same approach to the brain, since we are reaching a point where knowing the signal in the brain is potentially very helpful. The state of the brain is really the response, not the cause. It is giving us a signal as to how we might optimize its return to normality. That's a set of experiments that we are now trying to do.

Jack Kornfield: A similar diagnostic process is needed both in meditation teaching and in insight therapy. When people come in to see a teacher, they present specific and unique difficulties, traumas, problems with circumstances in their life, or struggles with their mind and personality. Skillful teaching requires a subtle evaluative process to sense what particular intervention out of the many practices will be most helpful to a given individual. For example, for people with powerful self-critical and judgmental thoughts, a necessary part of meditation instruction will be teaching them how to work with these thoughts. If we don't attend to this problem, they can do all kinds of other practices, but those self-critical patterns will keep repeating, "You're not doing it right," and as a consequence, the other practices they are engaging in may be quite ineffective.

Jan Chozen Bays: I want to suggest that we study an intervention that I call media fasting. As I said, we're not designed as an organism to take in the suffering of the whole world. We can only do that when we've undertaken Bodhicitta and a number of practice tools that help us take on that much suffering. In my own work with child abuse, I realized I needed, as an antidote to the suffering that I was taking in, to decrease the number of hours I was working in child abuse and increase my hours of meditation practice.

I have tried media fasting with some students, and it's been very helpful. We either nourish or assault the brain with what we take in through our senses. When we take in that much suffering and human cruelty, just as when we teach our youngest men to kill, to break the primary precept of all religion, we're doing a great wrong to the entire human organism. I don't watch television at the monastery, but when I stay at hotels, I do. My husband says, "Turn it off!" but it helps me understand what everybody else is taking in. All the violence that pours into our minds and hearts through television is really a terrible diet, especially for children. And then teaching our youngest people, our twenty- and thirty-year-olds who are going to inherit the world, to kill intentionally . . . Once you can intentionally kill another human being, then, of course, you can lie and steal and torture people and destroy property. It's downhill from there. So I think that the antidote of media fasting could be a very powerful treat-ment for our mental health, collectively and individually.

I have one other concern. We're doing fantastically well in treating conditions such as depression through our discoveries of medication and cognitive behavioral therapy and brain stimulation. It is truly wonderful that modern medicine can do this, but it sets up a subtle expectation that all suffering can eventually be relieved through technology and medical or biochemical means. I think we have to draw a clear distinction between relative relief of suffering and ultimate relief of suffering. The relative relief of suffering is rightly the purview of medicine, and its value is not to be underestimated. It is huge in its own right, and also because it may eventu-ally enable people to switch to what we might call the ultimate relief of suffering, which is the spiritual path.

Helen Mayberg: I certainly want to endorse what you are saying. The patients who have been treated by deep brain stimulation have helped me to understand this the best. Through the stimulation, we have helped them get to the point where they can participate in life and have some awareness that they didn't have before. I would not go so far as to say that the stimulation is the source of the awareness, but it brings the rest of the thinking brain, the self-aware brain, into balance so that these patients recognize they need to do something active. When we as physicians help our patients know that we are guides on a path, helping them get to a certain point and then handing them off to other teachers to continue the path and the guidance, then we both relieve suffering from a medical point of view and enhance well-being from a spiritual point of view. Patients need to have the expectation that we can get them back up to neutral.

Jack Kornfield: I'd like to see the next *Diagnostic and Statistical Manual of Mental Disorders* expanded beyond pathology. The upcoming revision should have a whole section on human potential and highly developed well-being. We should expand our vision, both individually and collec-tively. What is a wise society and what is a wise individual in a wise society? There are possibilities of profound inner peace, joy, creativity, and freedom—remarkable dimensions of mental health that all our collective work is pointing to.

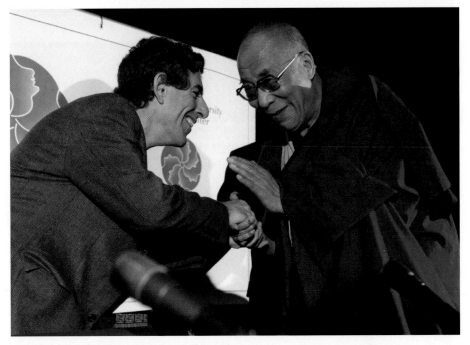

Richard Davidson welcoming His Holiness to the press conference preceding the meeting

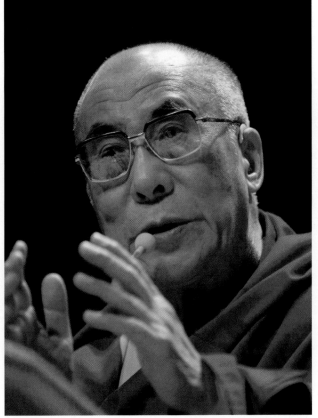

His Holiness making opening remarks from the lectern

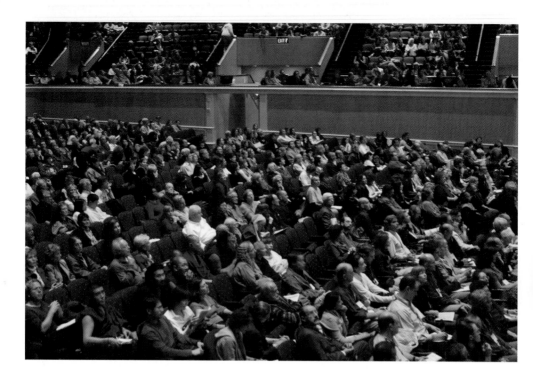

The audience

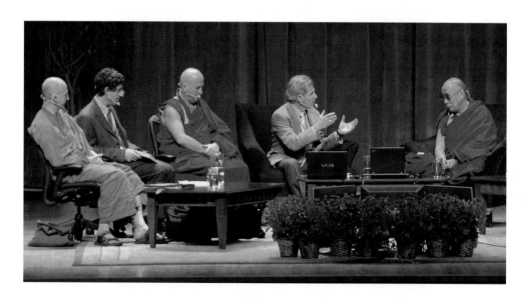

Jon Kabat-Zinn presenting to His Holiness, with Ajahn Amaro, Richard Davidson, and Matthieu Ricard listening

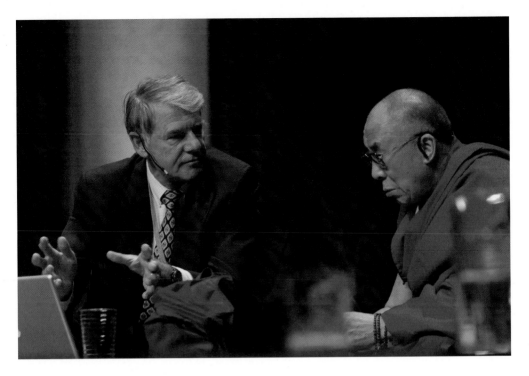

Wolf Singer presenting to His Holiness

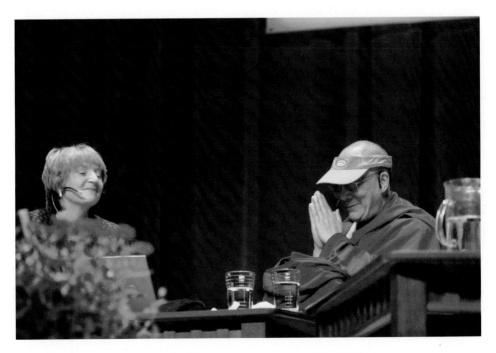

Helen Mayberg at the end of her presentation to His Holiness

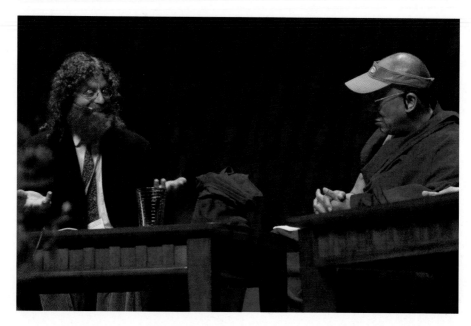

Robert Sapolsky with His Holiness

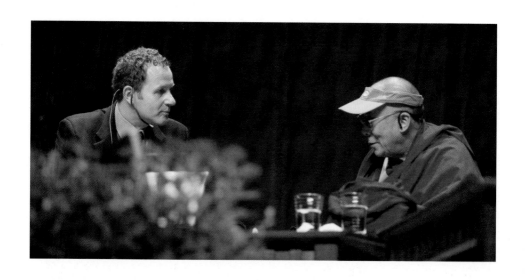

Zindel Segal with His Holiness

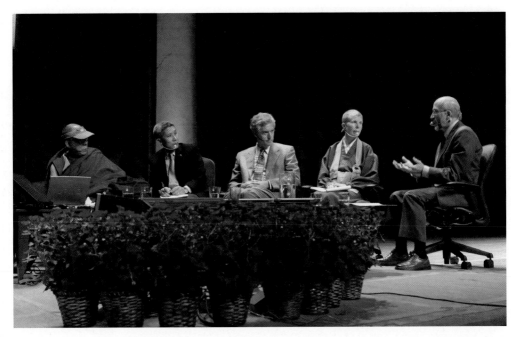

John Teasdale presenting to His Holiness, with Thupten Jinpa, Alan Wallace, and Jan Chozen Bays listening

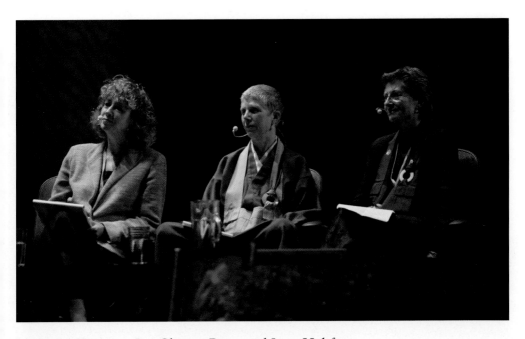

Margaret Kemeny, Jan Chozen Bays, and Joan Halifax

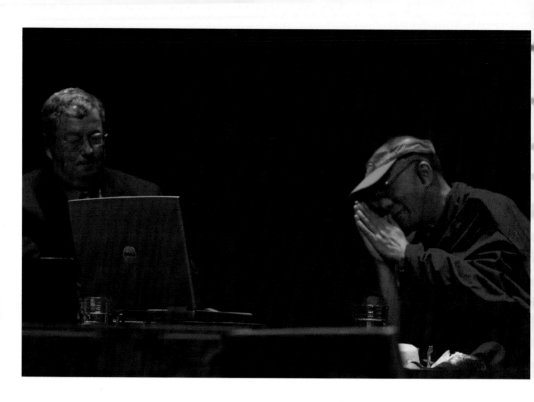

John Sheridan completes his presentation

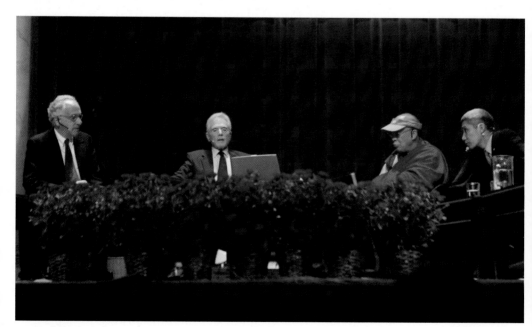

Ralph Snyderman presenting to His Holiness in the final session, with Ben Shapiro and Thupten Jinpa listening

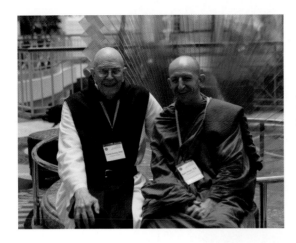

Father Thomas Keating
and Ajahn Amaro

Sharon Salzberg

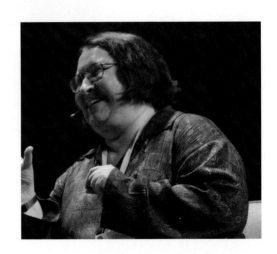

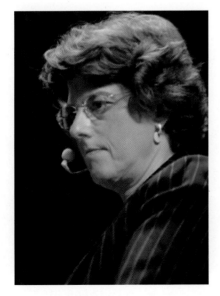

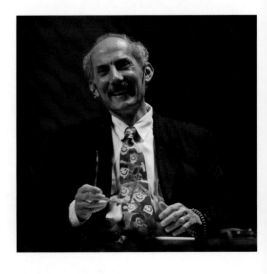

Esther Sternberg

Jack Kornfield

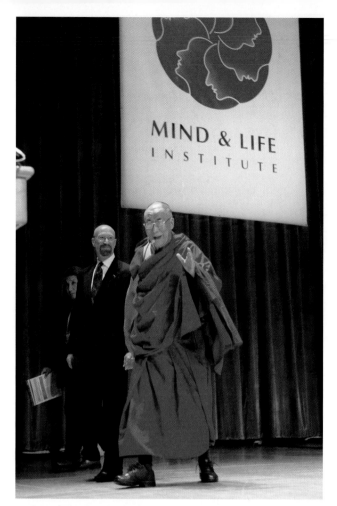

Adam Engle leads His Holiness offstage

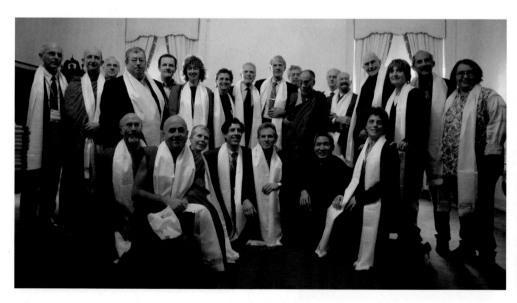

The entire group following session five. The white scarves, called *katas* in Tibetan, are a traditional gift of gratitude and blessing from His Holiness

Zindel Segal: To follow up on what Jack said, a lot of the way we identify emotional problems is by considering them as episodes. Something starts, you have a difficult time, then it ends, and you're back to being who you were. But if you look at the actual trajectory over people's lives, they have many episodes that start and stop. For some people with depression, they never actually pull out of it completely and continue to have difficulties in a low-grade way.

We are now starting to consider these not as episodes but as chronic problems that require different treatments from just fixing an episode. We can encourage people to practice lifelong ways of looking after themselves: mental training, even when they are not symptomatic; lifestyle changes such as exercise, even when they don't necessarily need to lose weight. These are examples of taking responsibility for one's own care. Meditation training is a very important part of that, along with other approaches that don't necessarily need the presence of an illness to be of benefit.

Jon Kabat-Zinn: That relates to what Alan was saying about an attitudinal shift. Your whole life can change in relationship to exercise or diet, for example. It's not like "Now I'm on a diet," but rather "This is simply the way I eat and the things I choose to nourish myself with," including the diet of what comes in through your eyes and your ears, through television, through the newspaper, and through your relationships.

John Teasdale: I see a tension between what we might do as meditation teachers—when individuals come to us whom we have the luxury of knowing personally—and what we may have to consider at a public health level. If we take seriously the idea that millions of people out there could potentially benefit, then we don't have that luxury. How can we creatively work with that tension? Clearly one way is Jon's approach with mindfulness-based stress reduction, where you do actually use a one-size-fits-all approach.

Jon Kabat-Zinn: With subtle modifications for all, and each.

John Teasdale: Yes, but basically that's the model. It seems to me that this tension is one we could very fruitfully live with, by somehow hanging on to the richness and wisdom that come from teaching individuals and funneling that in a way that could be delivered to help the millions of people who could benefit.

Jon Kabat-Zinn: Part of the beauty of this kind of dialogue is that we're beginning to see that multiple approaches are required to deal with the intrinsic heterogeneity of disease, or of mind states and brain states even within one disease. As His Holiness suggested, a salient feature of our species is that we are all so different and yet, at the same time, so similar.

The question is, Can we actually design interventions that can be continually more finely tuned by the practitioners themselves as they continue to develop along the trajectory of potential well-being? In my experience, MBSR and MBCT do offer that possibility and thus combine the generic and the specific, and can function on a large-scale public health level to potentially affect the lives of millions. As clinicians and as teachers, can we develop qualities of sensitivity, beyond the normal, baseline sensitivity, for a more profound way of seeing and being that might resonate with similar capacities and qualities in other people, in our patients for instance? In doing so, can we recognize both their suffering and their genius or true nature, their capacity to recognize something in themselves that is already okay, already whole?

Jan Chozen Bays: One of the first books that came out about the use of medication for depression was *Listening to Prozac*.[82] As I read this book, I was struck by one patient who had been depressed all of her life before she went on medicine. She changed, and she said to the doctor, "This is really me. Now I am really me." And I thought, how did she know that? Many people have that experience in meditation: "Ah, this is the true me, the real me!"

So I became curious—if we develop our technology so that people can change their state of mind with medication or by turning a dial on a stimulator, what will they choose? Will they choose to be a little sad because that's familiar? Will they choose neutral because it's balanced? Or will they choose happy? A psychiatrist told me that she allows her patients to change their medication by themselves, and they choose happy. That fits with Your Holiness's idea that everyone seeks happiness.

INTERLUDE
PRECEDING SESSION 4

Between the morning and midafternoon sessions, HH Dalai Lama visited the president of the United States at the White House. In this interlude, moderated by Richard Davidson, Alan Wallace offers an eloquent and incisive presentation on the Buddhist science of human flourishing, focusing on three themes: social flourishing in relation to society and the natural environment, psychological flourishing by cultivating four aspects of mental balance, and spiritual flourishing by gaining experiential insight into the nature of awareness itself. Afterward the meeting shifts to taking questions from the audience.

Richard Davidson: We have a wonderful treat this afternoon. Alan Wallace, a board member of the Mind and Life Institute, was a Buddhist monk for more than a decade before he returned to the United States and received his PhD from Stanford University in religious studies. Alan has been central to the Mind and Life Dialogues since their inception in 1987. He has also been a collaborator, a partner, a translator, and a person who has inspired, challenged, and provoked us in our research.

The monks living in the hills around Dharamsala that we initially visited when we first began this work with Francisco Varela more than a decade ago were people Alan was intimately acquainted with during his time as a monk in India. Were it not for the trust that those practitioners had in Alan as a colleague, we never would have been able to start this research. It is with a deep bow of gratitude that I introduce Alan, who will talk about the Buddhist science of human flourishing.

ALAN WALLACE *The Buddhist Science of Human Flourishing*

Traditional Buddhist meditative practices are designed not only to alleviate temporary pain and suffering, but to cultivate eudaimonic well-being, or human flourishing. This is done in an integrative fashion that includes the transformation of one's way of viewing reality, practices of meditation, and the cultivation of an ethical, altruistic way of life. By such means, one cultivates social well-being by way of ethics, psychological well-being by way of meditation, and spiritual well-being by way of contemplative insight. In the modern world, science is often presented as the sole means of acquiring knowledge of the natural world. Although science has achieved great triumphs regarding the objective world of matter and energy, Buddhist theories and practices of meditation have much to offer in terms of understanding the nature and potentials of consciousness and the cultivation of human flourishing.

Thus far, when we've spoken of the science of meditation, this has quite clearly implied the scientific study of meditation—its impact on the brain and health, the clinical applications of a particular form of meditation, mindfulness practice, and its multiple benefits in a myriad of fields. We could also ask, "What about the Buddhists? How do they use meditation?" Clearly, as we've seen from this dialogue, it has not been used traditionally to alleviate clinical depression or physical distress. So I'd like to address a Buddhist science of meditation, what His Holiness the Dalai Lama often speaks of as a Buddhist mind science, especially in terms of its role in achieving ever-deepening experiences of human flourishing.

I'm speaking now from a very specific tradition. Buddhism is twenty-five hundred years old and has been assimilated in a myriad of cultures—in Korea, Afghanistan, Mongolia, southeast Asia, and so on. There is no way I could possibly speak for all of the many schools, so I'll address this topic of a Buddhist science of meditation specifically from the Nalanda tradition, a current of Buddhism that His Holiness has often alluded to as being very relevant to the modern world.

Nalanda was a great monastic university that had its golden era about one thousand to fifteen hundred years ago. In the fifth century of the

Common Era, for example, it was a very well-established university with a student body of about ten thousand students, a faculty of about one thousand, and a central library eleven stories high. They studied five major and five minor fields of knowledge, not just Buddhism. They studied multiple spiritual, philosophical, and epistemological traditions, meditation and poetry, performing arts . . . The list went on and on. It was truly a university and a magnet for students from all over Asia.

From about the eighth to the thirteenth century, Nalanda was one of several monastic universities in India to which generations of Tibetans came. They migrated over the Himalayas to receive Indian Buddhist civilization—not just a religion, a philosophy, or a set of meditations, but really a civilization. It took them about five hundred years to bring it to Tibet. About the time they finished, something like a genocide took place in India, and those monasteries were all wiped out. The Nalanda tradition was preserved and developed for centuries since then in Tibet. The recent tragedy in Tibet was a great setback, but the same monasteries have been reestablished, some of them in India, and to my delight some have actually been reestablished in Tibet itself.

I'd like to begin my central topic with a quote from the Dalai Lama: "I believe that the very purpose of our life is to seek happiness. Whether one believes in religion or not, whether one believes in this religion or that religion, we all are seeking something better in life. So, I think, the very motion of our life is towards happiness."[83] This view is not unique to the Dalai Lama. It's characteristic of the Buddhist tradition as a whole and is found in Christian and other spiritual traditions as well: that the very meaning of life is the pursuit of happiness. It's kind of a happy thought.

But this raises the question of what kind of happiness. When Augustine, Aquinas, the Buddha, the Dalai Lama, and so many of the great sages of human history speak of happiness being the very meaning of life, what are they referring to? There is a convergence on this theme in the thinking of classical Greece, Buddhism, and modern psychology. They all distinguish what those in the field of positive psychology have come to call hedonic pleasure or hedonic well-being. The pursuit of happiness in this sense can be understood as the pursuit of pleasant stimuli. Things that make us happy in terms of hedonic pleasure are people we enjoy engaging with, an environment, a job, a medical plan, a certain amount of money in the bank, the number of children we have, good health, drugs in some cases—stimuli that provide us with or arouse us to a state of plea-sure, or at least a relief from suffering. It is the pursuit of pleasant stimuli and the avoidance of unpleasant stimuli.

The pursuit of happiness in these terms can be likened to the hunter-gatherer phase of civilizations, when people lived in small groups and foraged for sustenance, trying to find things that would give them plea-sure. As a metaphor, that's one orientation toward the pursuit of happiness: Go out into the world and find what makes you happy; then hold on to it for dear life.

I don't think that's what the Dalai Lama or any of the great sages from human history were primarily focusing on. What they had in mind was something that modern psychology has called eudaimonic well-being, from the Greek term *eudaimonia*, or "human flourishing," a way of being that provides one with a growing sense of fulfillment and meaning. I would define the pursuit of eudaimonic well-being as the integrative pursuit of inner happiness, a sense of well-being that springs from within, from the very quality of your heart, your mind, your awareness. The integrated pur-suit of inner happiness is not contingent upon pleasant things happening to you. It is integrated with the pursuit of truth and understanding the nature of reality. It is integrated with the pursuit of virtues that we all value, whether we're religious or not, qualities such as compassion, empa-thy, generosity, and so forth.

Eudaimonic well-being is not something you go out and forage for. It's not something you attain by finding the right person, the right setting, the great house, the great car. It's something that is cultivated, so I use the cultivator phase of human civilization as an analogue for that, where a larger group of people live together and invest in cultivating the soil rather than simply grabbing from nature. A smaller body of land can then sup-port a greater number of people.

The very word for meditation in Sanskrit, *bhavana*, means "to culti-vate." It doesn't mean anything esoteric, mystical, or occult. To meditate is to cultivate your heart, your mind. The Sanskrit and Pali word *citta*, or *sem* in Tibetan, means both "heart" and "mind." When you're cultivating com-passion, you're cultivating your citta. It's not a different part of your being.

A basic premise here is that a sense of wellness that springs from within is a symptom of a balanced, healthy, whole heart-mind—even without pleasant stimuli coming in from outside, even in the midst of completely neutral stimuli, just sitting quietly in a room, and also in the midst of unpleasant stimuli.

Is it possible to flourish in times of adversity? Is it possible to experience a sense of eudaimonic well-being, a sense of meaning and fulfillment, even in times of adversity or illness? We've heard a lot about how meditation may alleviate illness, which is wonderful. But what about those illnesses that won't go away? What about terminal illnesses, where the doctors say, "We can't help you. You're dying." Can we flourish in the face of death?

The Sanskrit term *dharma* means various things in various contexts, but when I asked one of my many Tibetan teachers long ago what dharma means, he said that dharma is the cultivation of a lasting state of well-being that arises from within, and the alleviation of suffering by overcoming the inner causes of suffering. It's the pursuit of genuine, eudaimonic well-being.

By the time Nalanda was founded more than fifteen hundred years ago, it was already drawing on a well-ripened tradition. The Buddha lived twenty-five hundred years ago, so they were already drawing not only on the realization, the experience, and the teachings of the Buddha himself, but on a thousand years of philosophers, contemplatives, and scholars of various sorts. They were drawing from an already ancient Buddhist civilization. There was also a rich contemplative heritage that preceded the Buddha, especially in training attention, and he drew from practices that had been developed generations before him. So the Nalanda tradition has a powerful intellectual heritage to it, empirical and interdisciplinary, but all oriented around dharma, the cultivation of genuine eudaimonic happiness or, as His Holiness calls it, liberation.

The framework for this richly textured, multifaceted practice entails three components. One is theory, or worldview. A theory is always a way of viewing reality from a perspective, whether it's a religious, philosophical, or scientific position. Your position always stands outside of your theory. Buddhist theory, for example, is a way of viewing reality that stems from ever-deepening contemplative experience, and also furthers one's own empirical inquiry.

A lot of Buddhist theory seems quite alien to the scientific worldview, so it's very easy to regard it as a metaphysical view. For example, when we're talking about the clinical applications of meditation, we'll say, "Let's set aside the metaphysical issues." But the word "metaphysical" is interesting, isn't it? *Meta*physical has the implication of being beyond physical, and also not empirical, not experiential. That statement comes from a position; it's not a statement from nowhere. It's based on the four hundred years since the scientific revolution, which was primarily physical in orientation. Copernicus did not direct his attention inward to explore the domain of consciousness, but outward to celestial phenomena. For the first three hundred years, scientific attention was focused almost entirely outward.

The scientific study of the mind didn't begin until about three hundred years after Copernicus. From about 1870 to 1900, scientists tried to develop an empirical approach to understanding mental phenomena, which they called introspection. It didn't do very well. By about 1910, they gave up trying to deal with subjective phenomena—they recognized they were no good at this—and behaviorism took over. Behavior is physical; we can deal with that. Now we have cognitive psychology, a lot of very sophisticated ways of studying the mind by way of behavior, and this glorious neuroscience, which studies mental phenomena by way of their neural correlates. But the fact that we tried introspection scientifically for thirty years, were terrible at it, and stopped doesn't necessarily mean that nobody else did any better.

Over the course of twenty-five hundred years, the Buddhist tradition never developed a theory of the brain, let alone a science of the brain. There's a good reason for that. As you hone your attention skills and become an adept with ten thousand or even forty thousand hours of training and introspection, exploring dimension upon dimension of the mind, unveiling layers and layers of the subconscious, the one thing you don't find, apparently, is the brain. You can't probe introspectively so deeply into your subconscious, in such a subtle fashion into the nature of mental processes, that you discover the hippocampus or the amygdala or the limbic area or the prefrontal cortex. It just doesn't come up. Buddhism has very elaborate, sophisticated theories about the nature of the mind and nothing about the brain. However, Buddhists got very good at the sophisticated, rigorous, highly trained, introspective study of mental phenomena.

So from a Buddhist perspective, His Holiness and the traditional Buddhists, including the monks here in the audience, are taking what the scientists say about the brain on faith. I think it's very well-deserved faith, and it's faith that I share. But from the Buddhist perspective, unless you're willing to put in many years of rigorous, sustained training in neuroscience, until that faith turns into knowledge, all that we've been hearing about the brain is outside of experience. It's "metamental"—that's the Tibetan word for metaphysical, translated back into English.

After all, what is metaphysical? It's what science hasn't been able to study yet. In the late nineteenth century, the nature of atoms was metaphysical. Chemists and physicists had their theories, but it was metaphysical because there were no empirical tests to determine which, if any, of these theories were right. The technology wasn't there. It is easy for us, dwelling in the fishbowl of Western civilization, to think that metaphysical is an ontological category that's somehow out there, hovering in midair. Is what is metaphysical for us necessarily metaphysical for everybody else? Maybe not. Maybe twenty-five hundred years of first-person inquiry have made some discoveries that seem metaphysical become purely empirical in the Buddhist tradition. They're metaphysical only insofar as you can't detect them with the instruments of technology.

Theory is the framework that stems from and supports one's spiritual practice. Then there's the second component, the meditation itself. In a Buddhist science of meditation, this is the cutting edge, the empirical probe. Meditation includes practices for transforming the mind, investigating the world of experience, and investigating the nature of the mind and its relationship with the body and with the environment. Thirdly, there's conduct. There are ways of life that are conducive to and support the cultivation of heart and mind, and there are ways of life that are detrimental to meditation. The theory, meditation, and conduct are all profoundly interwoven. They are mutually interdependent, and all three are critical.

As Ajahn Amaro pointed out earlier, the essentials of Buddhist practice consist of three parts: ethics, practice or mind training, and wisdom. Ethics is the foundation: a way of life that brings about social and also environmental flourishing, so that we can live in harmony with our natural environment as well as with human populations. Without ethics there's nothing; then you have anarchy, chaos, and misery.

On the basis of ethics—the foundation, I think, of all spiritual practice and certainly all Buddhist practice—there's a whole genre of practice that comes under the rubric of samadhi, which means "focused attention."

More broadly, it has to do with mental balance, with developing exceptional levels of mental health. This gives rise to psychological flourishing, to becoming exceptionally sane. And then, on that basis, one uses one's exceptionally sane, balanced, focused attention for the cultivation of wisdom. It's in the cultivation of wisdom that one finds the deeper level of eudaimonia, and in that realm of spiritual flourishing we find the liberation that His Holiness alluded to.

This is really just a brief overview. Each of these three areas can be seen as a science, taken purely empirically with no burden of dogma, no belief system that you must adopt. In his book *Ethics for the New Millennium*,[84] His Holiness has written with tremendous eloquence and depth about a Buddhist science of social flourishing based on ethical behavior. What kinds of behavior are conducive to one's own and others' environmental, social, psychological, and spiritual flourishing? What types of behavior undermine one's own and others' eudaimonic well-being? It's a whole science, and Buddhism has a great deal to say about it.

There's a Buddhist science of psychological flourishing, an extraordinary amount of material on mental balance, with dozens and dozens of meditative practices. There's tremendous diversity of different types of meditative training, some oriented toward exploration and investigation, some toward transformation or balancing. One aspect of psychological flourishing is conative balance, which relates to desire and intention. How do we cultivate desires that are conducive to our own and others' well-being? How do we gradually let go of, or attenuate, those desires, volitions, and motivations that are destructive to our own and others' well-being? That in itself is a whole science, and it requires metaconation, an awareness of what types of desires and intentions are arising in our minds.

Then there's the very rich area of attentional balance—starting from ADHD on up to the highest levels of samadhi, overcoming attentional imbalances of deficit and hyperactivity. There's an extraordinarily rich genre of theory and practice around attention, about which we have almost nothing in the modern West. It's a tremendous opportunity for collaboration, as in the Shamatha Project.

Psychological flourishing also includes cognitive balance. Are there times when we superimpose on reality our own projections, hopes, and unfounded fears and get into a lot of trouble by conflating our projections with reality? Are there times where we're simply AWOL on reality? As Jon likes to say, if you're not practicing mindfulness, you're practicing mindlessness. If reality is kicking you in the nose and you don't see it, a cognitive deficit might be the problem. Cognitive balance implies being present with what's going on, seeing it clearly and vividly.

Affective balance is another tremendously rich area of psychological flourishing. It does not mean getting into some steady, dronelike state of emotional equilibrium, but rather the buoyancy, lightness, and resiliency of emotional health. There are times of grieving and times of joy, but not times of neurosis, psychosis, or fixation in affective imbalances.

Finally, we have the Buddhist science of spiritual flourishing, which is frankly what Buddhism is ultimately about. The highly developed attention skills of samadhi are used as a telescope for the mind, becoming a very focused, stable, clear, vivid, malleable, and supple way of attending to a myriad of phenomena—potentially any type of phenomena, but specifically mental phenomena. So first we develop the tool, the telescope of refined attention. We then use that ability to explore the very nature of consciousness, the phenomenal experience of consciousness and its relationship to the universe at large. In so doing, we overcome the obscurations, afflictions, and imbalances of the mind, but we also cultivate the full potential of consciousness, tapping the deepest wellsprings of our own flourishing, knowing reality insofar as it can be known, by direct experience and the cultivation of virtue.

As I view my own civilization, it strikes me that in our modern world, these three pursuits—the pursuit of happiness, the pursuit of truth in understanding reality, and the pursuit of virtue—are often seen as unrelated. The advertising industry is banking on that. They'll sell you happiness—don't worry about truth—and the clear implication is that happiness has nothing to do with virtue. Science has an enormous amount to do with truth, but it often doesn't address the deeper issues of human flourishing or its relation to ethics. That could be a problem. When I try to envision a meaningful life, these are the three qualities that strike me as being essentially meaningful. Integrating them is also essential. To a very large extent, they've fallen apart, and I think the results are disastrous. The twentieth century witnessed exponential growth of knowledge and power. It was a glorious century for science and technology, and a disastrous century in terms of man's inhumanity to man—and I do emphasize the gender—and the degradation of our environment. How could we know so much and be so powerful, and yet treat each other so horribly and so savage our environment?

There needs to be some healing here. I see this time of crisis as a time of enormous opportunity for a collaboration between the scientific study of meditation and the contemplative study of the mind. By bringing together the great contemplative traditions of the world, not just Buddhism, with the scientific tradition—not dogma versus dogma, but empiricism wedded with empiricism—we may be able to help reintegrate, to reintroduce sanity and wholeness, allowing the brain of our global community to work together in synchrony to heal problems that are no longer localized. These are not just America's problems or Tibet's problems. We'll work together to reintegrate the natural sciences and humanities, and other types of polarities of which we are all very vividly aware, to heal ourselves as individuals, to heal our country, to heal our planet. I think there is great promise.

INTERLUDE DIALOGUE

Before the afternoon session gets under way, there is a period devoted to taking questions from the audience. Those responding are Ajahn Amaro, Richard Davidson, Jon Kabat-Zinn, Father Keating, Helen Mayberg, Matthieu Ricard, Zindel Segal, and Wolf Singer.

Jon Kabat-Zinn: This is a time to respond as best we can to some questions from the audience. Here is one: "Neurofeedback, also known as EEG biofeedback, is a powerful intervention process for regulating affect. Can anyone speak to this? It is as powerful as meditation and tremendously increases peace." Wolf, since you mentioned feedback in brain synchronization, perhaps you could take a first stab at the whole question of feedback from what we know that the brain is doing.

Wolf Singer: As I pointed out yesterday, it is possible to upregulate the activity of selected brain areas, even though the subject doesn't know which area has been picked by the experimenter. So it is possible to activate brain areas intuitively, by trial and error. In the same way, it is possible to influence the frequency spectrum of the electrodes' oscillatory activity in selected frequency bands. For example, if one plays back to the subject the amount of power in the alpha frequency band of around ten hertz, the subject, through trial and error, finds out how to increase the percentage of alpha waves produced per unit time.[85]

In the case of alpha feedback, this goes along with interior feeling states. The subjects feel relaxed. As far as I know, this has not been tried in higher frequency bands, partly for technical reasons. It would be tempting to assume that a Western shortcut to meditation could pick out the right frequencies and the right electrodes and have the subjects learn to produce those brain states without going through painful meditative practices!

It is doubtful that this is possible. We know that learning requires focused attention and an interplay with internal reward systems. In experiments with functional magnetic resonance imaging where subjects learn to activate selected brain centers, what we would have expected does not happen. Subjects have no feelings whatsoever, even if they activate centers that are known to be intimately involved in the production of emotions. So it's an open question.

Matthieu Ricard: There's also a kind of introspective self-feedback. When an emotion comes to mind, we are usually carried off by it and don't see the effect until afterward. But you can get immediate feedback by very finely examining your state of mind when you feel compassion or when anger arises. You can observe very minutely what the nagging effect of jealousy is. In a way, it's a kind of feedback if you can lucidly look at an emotion as a phenomenon, not identifying with it, but clearly seeing how dealing with it either increases or decreases it.

Richard Davidson: I think it's critical at this stage in our science to be humble about what we know and don't know. Although we have found certain neural correlates of certain aspects of particular meditation practices, this doesn't mean that these correlates necessarily represent the key elements of change that occur in the production of these states. It would be of interest to do neural feedback studies and assess the corresponding introspective accounts, but I also am humbled by the complexity of what we are studying. The methods we're using are much more precise than they were a decade ago, but they are still very crude. There is so much basic research that needs to be done to assess which signals are most closely associated with length of practice and how much a person changes over time and in what ways. Those issues are still unclear, so I think we should be cautious about prematurely rushing to apply neurofeedback technology.

Ajahn Amaro: The basic paradigm that the Buddha used for any spiritual methodology is "Does it reduce suffering or not?" Regardless of the theoretical background, what's the effect? So one of my basic maxims is "If it works, it's the right thing." I've never used biofeedback—externally—but if people find that it actually helps reduce suffering, makes them feel more harmonious, or allows them to understand life better, then it's all well and good. The quality that Matthieu was referring to is called *vimamsa* in the Pali language. It's the fourth element of the iddhipada, or "the four bases of success": interest, energy, contemplation, and reviewing or feedback. That kind of reviewing, considering the results of what you've done, is considered a crucial element in succeeding at any kind of task. Without feedback, whether internal or with little blinking lights, you can't really tell what the results are of what you're doing.

Richard Davidson: This next question is one the contemplatives may be particularly suited to answer. This person asks, "Have there been any observed detrimental effects of meditation, such as loss of sense of self in a negative way? What are the potential dangers of this kind of meditation? Examining our minds can sometimes be a painful experience."

Alan Wallace: "Meditation" is a broad term. It just means messing around with your mind in a sustained way, and the mind, like the nervous system or the brain, is very delicate. If you are meditating on your own, making it up as you go, you might be lucky. But if you do any type of meditative practice intensively, it's like setting out on a ship. If you're just one degree off, you can wind up hundreds of miles away from where you intended to go.

Over the last thirty-five years that I've been involved in this, I've encountered a number of people who have run into very deep psychological problems, including psychosis. Usually it occurred when they were not practicing under the guidance of a skillful, knowledgeable, and compassionate teacher. An open and trusting relationship with a teacher is a great safety net. If one is meditating ten or fifteen minutes a day, the chances of damage are small. If you push that up to ten or twelve hours a day, you want some very skillful guidance and a lot of intelligence in the practice.

Father Keating: I think there is a hazard to almost anything. You can walk down the street and be hit on the head with a brick. Meditation isn't any more hazardous than any other form of living, as far as I can see. I think it's more hazardous not to meditate. It's like driving down a road that is full of potholes: you can decide to pull over to the side of the road and wait until the county fixes all the potholes, or you can go down the road as best you can and try to stay out of them.

Meditation is full of mistakes, heartaches, and boring moments, and the feeling of getting nowhere. It's doing it every day, preferably twice a day, that makes all the difference. Then it becomes a divine therapy that does two things. It spontaneously affirms our basic goodness, hence addressing the whole panorama of low self-esteem that is epidemic in Western culture. The other thing meditation addresses is the unconscious and all the repressed emotional junk of a lifetime. That repressed material is warehoused in the body and causes all kinds of problems.

Perhaps the greatest step toward happiness that we can make is to recognize that happiness and pleasure are not the same thing. There's an enormous distinction between the two. Pleasure is the gratification of our instinctual needs. As infants we mistake that for happiness because we don't have any choice yet of mental or spiritual possibilities. The kind of information we learn by allowing unconscious and repressed material, emotional trauma from the past, addictive behavior, and negative motivation to come to consciousness and be evacuated is so important. The body uses the deep rest of meditation as permission to evacuate what shouldn't be stored in our nervous system or in our muscles. It's one of the great sources of health that meditation provides.

Matthieu Ricard: Once I met a young person who said, "I don't want to look in my mind because I am afraid of what I will find there." I mentioned that to His Holiness, who said, "But it's more interesting than going to a movie! There's so much happening in there. It's so interesting!"

People often hesitate to investigate their minds, and to investigate the inner mechanisms of happiness and suffering. What's surprising is how little time or concern we have for understanding how our minds work, even though we deal with our minds from morning to evening. That's what determines the quality of every instant of life. We spend so much effort and time on education, getting a job, beauty, fitness, and so on, and so little time taking care of that "spoiled brat" of a mind, you could say, that creates so much trouble all day long.

Jon Kabat-Zinn: Here's another question from the audience: "It's often difficult to motivate highly depressed people to meditate in isolation, when working in individual therapy, for instance. Is the social support from sangha in MBCT also part of your work? Is that part of why you see good results?" That raises an issue that Jack Kornfield brought to the fore this morning: how different elements contribute to the context in which one is investigating one's own experience. Put otherwise, how do we create appropriate holding environments to optimize any experience of meditation?

Zindel Segal: It's a very good question. Once again, we need to distinguish between people who are very depressed and those who have come out of a depression and are looking to stay well, though they may have minor symptoms of depression and are still skating on thin ice. These therapies are very brief, just eight weeks of training with daily practice, and it's over. People complain that what's missing is a secular sangha that can be accessed in a very conventional, convenient manner. That is hard to find.

In the hospital, we offer a monthly or even weekly group for people to sit together. But many people don't want to return to the hospital. They want to integrate this into an ongoing view of their own wholeness. It reminds me of the community mental health centers they used to have, where people could just drop in. We need something like that, a way for people to feel connected and take advantage of the supports that a community sitting together can provide. On a large scale, it relates to what John Teasdale said about disseminating this work more widely. Some sort of resource like that is required.

Helen Mayberg: Even without considering meditation, as patients recover from depression and reach a point of being ready to engage with others, family becomes essential. Patients, like everyone, need feedback that they are in an environment with people who care about them. Part of recovery is realizing that you're not alone, and that perspective needs reinforcement, whether it's facilitated by a meditation teacher or a physician.

Even for our patients with brain stimulators, it's clear that although the treatment removes the noise and intensity of the illness, what ensures patients really recover and are engaged in the community is feedback from others. The mindfulness approach is fantastic because you don't have to think about why you were sick in order to engage with focused attention in a way that reinforces your path to recovery.

Matthieu Ricard: Helen, last week at Stanford, when we both attended the conference on the subject of suffering, you mentioned the sense of connectedness that comes back when the patients are improving.

Helen Mayberg: I think that is one of the most dramatic changes we see. One patient was so aware of the depths of her illness. It was not just that she couldn't sleep or eat or work, but that when she held her children, she couldn't feel them. Some physicians consider that nearly psychotic. In fact, the ultimate deprivation of the illness is how it interferes with the ability to connect with others.

The awareness of connecting with the physicians that this patient experienced when undergoing brain stimulation in the operating room was quite striking for her, because lack of connection was such a profound aspect of her illness. It was important to transmit to her family that she experienced that and was able to express it at this early stage of recovery. Not all patients realize that this is what they're missing. That particular patient taught me how profound it is. It isn't just about yourself and your pain; it's also about being free to interact with those around you. That's the essence of what we all search for, whether we're sick or well.

Matthieu Ricard: Zindel, I know you don't completely agree with this, but someone mentioned that the incapacity to feel and to give love in deep depression is one of the main obstacles to recovery.

Zindel Segal: I don't disagree that it is phenomenologically very real. The way I understand it is that people are undecided as to whether they deserve to receive love from others, so they may distance themselves in their own minds from people praising them or even wanting to connect with them. That is a very big obstacle to them loving themselves enough to step out of what they're doing to themselves.

Matthieu Ricard: It also has to do with identifying in oneself a potential for change. When people hate themselves, this is reinforced when they think there's no room for change. Perhaps recognizing that there is in fact potential for transformation could help.

SESSION 4

CLINICAL RESEARCH 2: MEDITATION AND PHYSICAL HEALTH

As scientific research establishes that many "physical" diseases are modulated by psychological processes such as stressful life events and emotions, the mechanisms underlying these interactions have become targets for scientific research. As the understanding of these mechanisms grows, the rationale for using meditation as an intervention for certain types of physical illnesses becomes more compelling and more solidly grounded in contemporary scientific research. This session, moderated by Esther Sternberg, showcases modern research on the application of meditation-based interventions to cardiovascular disease and to medical conditions that include a primary immune component.

Esther Sternberg: In the previous sessions we heard about mental processes and brain processes that occur in meditation and in mental states of suffering, such as depression. In the session with Dr. Sapolsky, we began to touch on stress and how the events that occur in the brain when we are under threat can potentially affect the body and physical health. In this session we're going to move that discussion further. We're going to delve much more deeply into how the brain's stress hormones, which are released when we are under threat, can affect the functioning of the heart and the immune system.

We're very fortunate to have with us two experts in the field: Dr. David Sheps and Dr. John Sheridan. David will speak first. He is the associate chair of cardiology at the University of Florida College of Medicine, and is going to be talking to us about how mental stress affects the heart.

DAVID SHEPS *Mindfulness-Based Stress Reduction and Cardiovascular Disease*

Psychological stress can markedly decrease blood flow to the heart, dramatically elevating the risk of sudden cardiac death. This talk describes the protocol of an ongoing NIH-funded study of the impact of mindfulness-based stress reduction on blood flow responses to mental stress in cardiac patients using cardiac imaging, and on their quality of life. (Editors' Note: The study has been completed. However, for various reasons, the data has not yet been analyzed, so the results remain unknown at the time of publication.)

My talk has to do with how the negative mind states that we term "psychological stress" affect the heart. I'll describe a study now in process where we hope to reverse the deleterious effects of this physiological reaction through training in MBSR. Thinking about the effects of stress on the body sometimes brings to mind a cartoon I once saw showing a patient with his hair standing straight up and the doctor saying, "I suspect your problem is stress related." Unfortunately, most of the time physicians have no idea whether an individual patient is under stress unless they ask. Most patients don't present with their hair standing on end, so it can be a real challenge for us. And just as stress is endemic in our culture, so too is heart disease. To underscore the magnitude of the problem, over twelve million people in the United States have coronary artery disease, and 335,000 people a year die suddenly of coronary artery disease. These are statistics from 2005.

A very important epidemiologic case control study of myocardial infarction, or heart attack, was done in fifty-two countries and published in *The Lancet*.[86] Called the INTERHEART study, it found that psychosocial stress is responsible for almost 40 percent of the risk of myocardial infarction. This is true worldwide, for males and females, and all different types of people. So it's a very big problem.

In a study where the coronary arteries of patients with coronary artery disease are injected with dye in a heart catheterization laboratory, we can see the narrowing of a diseased vessel. When the patient is asked to subtract seven from one hundred serially, that brief bit of mental stress totally cuts off the circulation.[87]

We know from epidemiologic or population studies that stress is bad for many individuals. When a disaster, such as an earthquake or a missile attack in war, causes high degrees of stress, there is an increased rate of heart attacks and sudden death in the population. This is a consistent finding. Other studies show that heart attacks are increased just by episodes of anger experienced by an individual.

To study this in the laboratory, we present either exercise or a mental stress stimulus, and then measure various markers of heart function, such as amount of blood flow to the heart, which we call perfusion. We can measure whether or not the patient has chest pain, abnormal wall motion, or pumping function, and we can do an electrocardiogram.

One type of stressor that we use in the laboratory is a public speaking task. While we take patients' blood pressure and electrocardiogram, we ask them to think about how they would react to a negative situation in daily life, such as a close relative being mistreated in a nursing home. The patient has two minutes to prepare a speech and three minutes to give a talk, and we film the speech. We also inject the patient with harmless material that accumulates in the heart according to blood flow.

This public speaking task creates an ischemia, a state of deficient blood supply in the heart, in 30 to 50 percent of patients with documented coronary disease.[88] Usually it is a silent ischemia, not associated with chest pain. Even the patient is not aware that this is happening. It occurs at a lower heart rate threshold than standard exercise testing, and it is often not detected by electrocardiogram markers in the laboratory. There are a number of mechanisms that might explain its occurrence. One is decreased blood flow in the large coronary vessels. Another is decreased blood flow in the smaller, microscopic vessels. A third is increased demand for oxygen due to large elevations in blood pressure, which are very common.

We did a study sponsored by the NIH several years ago, the Psychophysiological Investigations of Myocardial Ischemia (PIMI) study, that had a similar protocol.[89] That study looked at patients, both men and women, with documented coronary disease and abnormal exercise tests.

We measured the left ventricular pumping chamber response, or wall motion, as an indicator of stress-induced ischemia, and then we followed the patients for cardiac events.

We followed these patients for five years after this test, and those who had abnormal heart function during the speech stressor had a three times greater risk of dying over five years than patients who had normal function or no evidence of ischemia during the stressor.

So mental stress can cause heart patients to have ischemia, and this is not healthy. The next question is, How can we can treat this problem? We designed a study, funded by the National Heart, Lung, and Blood Institute, using mindfulness-based stress reduction to decrease mental stress in patients with this condition. We have 150 patients assigned to either MBSR, usual care, or an educational control where patients have the same hours of contact with an instructor as the MBSR group, but instead of learning MBSR, they are educated on risk factors and other things.

We selected MBSR because it is a widely used approach for stress reduction. It is very well standardized, and previous studies have shown that participants tend to maintain their positive outcomes for a good period of time afterward. In addition, the instructors are trained in a uniform way, so if we get good results from this study, it would be generalizable. When the study is completed, we hope to be able to answer three questions: First, does training in mindfulness meditation via MBSR improve the heart's response to stress in terms of stress-induced ischemia? Second, is there improvement in the heart rate response to daily life stress? And third, does MBSR improve mental health and quality of life in general? Right now we are in the middle of the study. We don't have any results yet, but we hope to have some good information in a few years.

Esther Sternberg: Now we will hear from Dr. John Sheridan, one of the pioneers in psychoneuroimmunology and the associate director of the Institute for Behavioral Medicine Research at Ohio State University. He will speak on the effects of stress on the immune system and address the question of whether stress can make you sick.

JOHN SHERIDAN *Neural-Immune Interaction*

> *Various forms of stress affect specific brain systems, and through alter-*
> *ations in these circuits, profound changes in immune function can*
> *arise. This talk presents an overview of modern research on the impact*
> *of different kinds of stress on specific immune processes and the mech-*
> *anisms through which these effects are produced. This body of research*
> *can illuminate the mechanisms by which meditation may influence*
> *diseases of the immune system.*

It's unusual for me as a scientist to come up on stage and not have the protection of my data, but I've been asked to give a more conceptual talk about the work I've been doing for the last fifteen years on how the immune system protects the body and how stress and neural factors affect immune function.

I will make three major points. I'm working in the world of the body, with the immune system, but the immune system is itself controlled by the brain. In recent years we've also realized that the body feeds back into the brain, so there is bidirectional communication. The brain talks to the body, and the body talks back to the brain. This is very significant in deal-ing with infectious challenges.

The second point I'm going to talk about is how stress influences the immune system, via the brain, and how that might increase susceptibility to infectious challenges. For example, when we have a deadline we are trying to meet, we may not make time to meditate or exercise, or to get enough sleep. What happens after we make that deadline? We might col-lapse with some sort of illness, often an infection of some kind.

My third point is that not all stressors are equal. Some have negative consequences, some have positive consequences, and my experience of a stressor may not be the same as your experience of that very same stressor. There are all sorts of elements at play, but ultimately I want to know how a person's perception of the environment influences his or her immune system, and therefore susceptibility to disease.

As an immunologist, I am interested in how bacterial and viral infections or tissue injury induce inflammation and an immune response, and how that response terminates the replication of the pathogen and resolves the infection. This process takes some days. Over the years we've come to understand that many factors—environmental, behavioral, and psychosocial—can influence how the immune system responds to infection. We call this discipline psycho-neuroimmunology. It investigates the interactions among the domains of behavior, endocrine function, and the immune system.

We know that stress can affect disease, and we know some of the mechanisms and the pathways that are activated. We also know that stress modulates the immune system, and we want to work out the mechanisms. In studies we've been doing in both humans and mice, we've been looking at which cells of the immune system are influenced by which products of the nervous and endocrine systems when you get stressed.

The immune system talks to the brain. For example, when you have an infection, macrophages move to the point of infection and express a whole series of new genes to make new proteins called cytokines, which are basically hormones. These cytokines get into the bloodstream and are carried to the brain, where they can then influence behavior. Yesterday, Robert Sapolsky discussed how stress reactions are necessary for survival. What we call illness behavior is part of this picture. Illness behavior is driven by the production of cytokines, which are made locally in the body but move to the brain.

These cytokines turn on specific regions of the brain, including regions involved in responding to stress. Bidirectional communication occurs as the brain recognizes those signals and activates the hypothalamic-pituitary-adrenal axis, or HPA axis. The HPA axis constitutes an important part of the neuroendocrine system that regulates many physiological processes, such as digestion, metabolism, immunity, and the response to stress. Ultimately, in response to stress, the HPA axis releases adrenocorticotropic hormone, which causes the release of glucocorticoids, such as cortisol. Glucocorticoids are steroids, which are powerful regulatory molecules. The glucocorticoid response plays a very important role in maintaining health. This kind of bidirectional communication—body to brain and brain to body—changes the pattern of glucocorticoid responding, which exerts tremendous effects on the expression of genes within immune cells. While all of this can be adaptive, these processes can be altered dramatically by chronic, unrelenting stress that goes on for days to weeks.

Robert Sapolsky mentioned that acute stress is stimulating, an activating process that may contribute to survival. In many instances, acute stress enhances the immune system. But when the stress is chronic, it tends to suppress immunity. In two human studies that we've done, we looked at whether an immune response can be influenced by chronic stress. With my colleagues Janice Kiecolt-Glaser, Ronald Glaser, and others at Ohio State, we examined the stress of being a caregiver. The spousal caregivers of individuals with Alzheimer's disease on average are about sixty-eight years of age and are involved with tremendously stressful care of their spouse twenty-four hours a day, seven days a week, for three years.[90]

We asked whether these individuals respond to a vaccination the same way that a matched control group does. We found that 70 percent of the individuals in the control group responded to the vaccine with a four-fold increase in antibody titer, which is significantly protective in neutralizing the virus. However, in the caregiver group, only around 35 percent responded at that level, which is a 50 percent reduction in the number of individuals responding in that way.

In summary, it looks like chronic stress does influence the ability to respond to a vaccine. We've done this now with hepatitis A,[91] hepatitis B,[92] and a streptococcal pneumonia vaccine.[93] If this observation holds up, it suggests that these individuals are at increased risk for infectious disease.

I had the good fortune a few years ago to meet Richie Davidson and Jon Kabat-Zinn. They asked me to be involved with them in a study using the same protocol to see if mindfulness meditation could influence responsiveness to a vaccine. We found small but statistically significant incremental increases in antibody responses in a workforce population who were given MBSR training.[94] We really need to repeat and extend this study, but it indicates that meditation can influence the brain-to-periphery communication in a beneficial way in terms of vaccinations.

The problem I have as an immunologist is that I'm very restricted in the sites that I can sample. I can take your blood and, if you're willing, a little piece of tissue on your skin, but I can't do much more than that. The real challenge in studying viral or bacterial infection is actually looking at all of the immune system, not just the response to being exposed to a vaccine. Looking at the whole immune system is much more complicated, and we can't do it in humans because we cannot infect individuals. So we've developed a number of animal models that combine well-established viral or bacterial infections with a number of different stress models. These stress models address the point that not all stressors affect the immune system equally. We can pick and choose how we modulate an animal's immune system by the application of a specific stressor, and then simply ask whether that animal is more or less susceptible to infection. You can see why we have to do this in animals, because we need to use live challenges.

One example is simple confinement stress. We take mice and isolate them from their mates in a tube overnight and then let them go. After a couple of nights we infect them with an influenza virus and look at what happens to their natural killer cell activity. Natural killer cells are a key component of our genetically inherited resistance to disease. They play a very important role in containing infection in the first two or three days. After we infect the animals, natural killer cell activity is a good way to measure their response to the infection. If we stress those animals for just a couple of days during infection, we can suppress the natural killer cell activity.

Because we are working with animals, we can do something more. We can ask which of the pathways between brain and body are sending the signals that suppress this response. We can pharmacologically treat the animals to block the glucocorticoids, or other signals such as opioids or catecholamines. Catecholamines, which are released by the sympathetic nervous system in response to stress, are known as the fight-or-flight hormones. In this case we used a restraint stress model in which activation of the hypothalamic-pituitary-adrenal axis leads to the production of opioids.

Opioids are hormones involved in the perception and suppression of pain, but they also suppress the natural killer cell response. If we block the opioid receptors, we can restore full natural killer cell response and restore the health of the animal. We've observed that when stress suppresses the natural killer cell response, this leads to more severe influenza infection. In this model, suppression of innate resistance by stress leads to enhanced disease.[95] The implication is that stress may lead generally to susceptibility to a number of different infectious microorganisms.

For the most part, everybody thinks stress is bad, if sometimes necessary for survival. So now I want to show you a model using social interaction, where stress leads to a positive benefit and actually enhances resistance to disease. Mice, like all mammals that live in groups, establish a hierarchy, which becomes a stable family. If we then add a large male intruder—like your dean or your chair coming to your office, for those of you who are academics—he disrupts the homeostasis in the cage. If you do this randomly on a couple of nights, the disruption is very stressful. The animals respond by activating all the stress hormones, and they also change their behavior.

After a single night of this stress, you can measure the behavior change and see an increase in anxiety. In addition to the behavioral change, you get an endocrine change: very high levels of glucocorticoids. Glucocorticoids are normally nature's most immunosuppressant substance and are also highly suppressive of most gene expression. In this case, however, the high level of glucocorticoids fails to suppress tumor necrosis factor and interleukin-1, cytokines that are involved in the inflammatory response. In these animals that we've challenged, we find that the social stress behavior increases the inflammatory response.

We then challenge them further with E. coli bacteria and measure the number of bacteria in circulation. The control mice get rid of the bacteria slowly but surely over a couple of hours, but the group that experienced social stress show increased clearance of the bacteria. These animals are more resistant to this bacterial infection as a consequence of the stressful interaction.[96] The implication is that this particular social stressor may enhance resistance to bacterial infection. However, we can't extrapolate easily between species, so I'm not going to project this from a mouse to a human, but there is a world of possibilities.

In summary, in humans and in animal models, bidirectional communication between the brain and the immune system is meaningful in terms of health. Not all stresses affect that communication in the same way or even the same direction. Some may actually be beneficial. We have a long way to go to understand the complex interactions that are occurring.

SESSION 4 DIALOGUE

In addition to HH Dalai Lama and the presenters, translators, and moderator, panelists for this session include Jan Chozen Bays, Richard Davidson, Joan Halifax, and Margaret Kemeny.

159

Esther Sternberg: Thank you, John and David, for this discussion of how all of those hormones and molecules that are released when we are exposed to many sorts of threats affect the body, the heart, and the immune system. From John we heard that stress hormones, the glucocorticoids, turn down immune cells' ability to fight infection. From David we heard how those stress effects can squeeze the coronary arteries, reduce blood flow to the heart, and increase risk of mortality. As small a stressor as subtracting seven from one hundred serially or speaking to an audience can have a profound effect on health.

At lunch we had a very lively discussion during which many of us were stressed over whether we should use the word "stress" when we talk to you, Your Holiness. As I understand it, in Tibetan there is no one word for stress in the sense that we use the word. I think that raises a very important question. We in the Western tradition are so grounded in objective, concrete thinking, defining health as only the absence of disease. We feel that we must relate everything to mechanism and how things work. This is wonderful, and this is how science has advanced, but how can we have a dialogue with you if we're using different terms? I would ask you then to comment on the fact that we do use different terms. We in Western medicine think about many different kinds of stress, social and physical. How do you think about stress? Is there such a thing as stress in your tradition?

HH Dalai Lama: The word "stress," as used in the clinical sense, has no exact Tibetan translation . . .

Thupten Jinpa: We were having a quiet discussion yesterday in the middle of the presentations, trying to figure out what the closest equivalent to the English term "stress" is in Tibetan, but there seems to be no equivalent term in Tibetan.

Esther Sternberg: I think that's a very important point, because if we are going to have a dialogue, the first thing we need to do is realize that we're speaking very different languages, not only in terms of English and Tibetan, but in terms of our conceptual framework. We keep trying to bring the conversation back to clinical applications—that's what the title of the meeting is—and the treatment of disease. Yet what we're all learning from you is that this isn't the goal in your tradition. I would ask you to expand on what the goal of meditation is from your perspective.

HH Dalai Lama: The objective of spiritual practice in the traditional context of Buddhism was well summarized by Ajahn Amaro in the framework of the three trainings: ethical discipline, cultivating concentration, which is the meditation practice, and, based upon that, cultivating insight.

At the initial stage, because some of our impulsive behavior is destructive and damaging, we need to find a way to restrain ourselves from engaging in these impulsive, destructive actions. This first stage of training is where we deliberately adopt a set of precepts or a code of life, which is the training in ethical discipline.

Since these impulsive, destructive behaviors really stem from a restless, undisciplined state of mind, we need to find a way of dealing with them directly. But our normal state of mind is so dissipated and unfocused that the mind cannot deal with mental problems immediately. Therefore one must first cultivate a degree of mental stability, an ability to focus. This is where the second training in concentration or meditation comes in.

On that basis, once we have a certain degree of stability, then we are able to use our mind, empowered with a focused attention, to deal with destructive emotions and habitual thought patterns. The antidote that overcomes the negative and destructive tendencies of the mind is insight.

Esther Sternberg: I'll try to extrapolate this then to the goal of this afternoon's session, which is to understand whether we can take those practices that are so well developed in your tradition and apply them to the problem that we call stress. I think what I'm hearing from you is that when we talk about stress, it's something that's happening to us; and when you talk about meditation, it's something that you are actively doing to train yourself.

HH Dalai Lama: Here we must understand how Buddhism views the essence of ethics. Ethical discipline is defined in terms of restraining not only from actions that are immediately harmful to others, but also from potentially harmful actions. When you engage in that level of training, at the heart of ethical discipline you are really responding to the environment. You abstain from harming others, and you try to live a life that is more heedful. Heedlessness is thought to be one of the core conditions that give rise to all sorts of destructive behavior.

In the training of concentration, and particularly in the third training, of insight, it becomes very specifically Buddhist. Each spiritual tradition might have different content insofar as their insights are concerned. Obviously for some people the monotheistic approach with the idea of a creator is much more effective. In Buddhist and some other ancient Indian systems of thought, there is no idea of a creator. So you enter into the very specific domains of different spiritual traditions.

What we are trying to do here, as we mentioned yesterday, is to focus on universal compassion or universal values. If the goal related only to some specific domain, there would be a lot of complications. It would be no use.

Esther Sternberg: We make life too complicated on our side, perhaps.

HH Dalai Lama: When you listen to the neuroscientific explanations, there is not just the brain, but so many parts of the brain, with so many sophisticated, complex names to each part.

Richard Davidson: Just like the Abhidharma.

HH Dalai Lama: Perhaps in the psychological domain, Buddhism has more terminology. Modern science mainly deals with physical or external things. We need that; modern science is very, very important. But in the meantime we also have experience and feeling. Ancient Indian thought dealt extensively with emotion and the mind. That is also useful; so we should combine these two things, up to a certain level. Then there's the next life, or nirvana! These are something of a specialty to the Buddhists. Whether there is heaven or hell, that is theistic business. It is not our business. I think it is better to have a noninterference policy!

Esther Sternberg: That's a hard line to follow. I'm going to ask Margaret Kemeny to take the responsibility of addressing this and bringing it back to a point of connection that we do have, which has to do with the self. Stress involves threats to the self, and how those threats can affect physical health. Margaret Kemeny is a professor of psychiatry and director of Health Psychology at the University of California, San Francisco. She is one of the pioneers in psychoneuroimmunology.

Margaret Kemeny: Your Holiness, I would like to shift the focus a bit, and I hope very much that you would be interested in talking about the Buddhist conception of self as well as the Buddhist conception of the social self. As I understand it, the two can be distinguished. I'm interested in hearing the Buddhist perspective on the self because there's a lot of evidence now that situations that threaten the sense of self can activate stress hormones and immunologic processes that can have a negative effect on health if activated chronically, as John Sheridan discussed. Threats to the sense of self seem to be reliable and powerful activators of these systems.

If you put people in a situation where they are performing a difficult task and are being evaluated by others, it can provoke these biological systems and cause emotions of anxiety and distress. It can cause people to feel negatively about themselves and to feel that others are reacting negatively to them. It can also cause self-conscious emotions, such as feelings of embarrassment, shame, and humiliation.

What's interesting is that not everyone shows these negative biological changes. The people who feel bad about themselves in that context, who feel embarrassed or humiliated or experience themselves as deficient, are the ones who show this biological change. I think we may be more vulnerable to these threats to our sense of self in our culture because of our focus on the individual rather than the group or collective. I wonder about the Buddhist view of the self and whether Buddhist notions of the self might increase our understanding of this vulnerability. For scientists, it would help to know how meditation and contemplative practices might decrease people's vulnerabilities in those situations. It would be so helpful to get more understanding of the Buddhist conception of the self.

HH Dalai Lama: The philosophical idea of no-self that you find in Buddhism is a very uniquely Buddhist concept. The reason why the understanding of no-self is given such importance is because of the recognition that the various problems of undisciplined states of mind are rooted in a false grasping at self. The Buddhist understanding of the mechanism by which we create all the afflictions in our mind and the problems that we run into is quite complex. The understanding is that our problems really stem from afflictions of the mind, which create an undisciplined, restless state. Within the spectrum of these different afflictions, there are some that are more affective, like attachment and hostility, and that can be directed to a specific object. They involve a particular way of relating to objects.

These afflictions are on the more manifest levels of gross consciousness, but other afflictions are thought to be much more deeply rooted. They are referred to as dysfunctional, belonging to a class of intelligence

163

rather than a more reactive, affective class. Underlying them is the false belief in self, or grasping at self. It is because of this that there is so much emphasis on understanding no-self—that there is no self postulated as eternal or absolute.

The Buddha talks about how the process of overcoming these afflictions takes place not in one instance of an awakening to no-self, when everything sort of falls apart. Rather, it is through a much more prolonged, gradual process, with many different factors coming together, that one can gradually overcome both intellectual, acquired afflictions and those that are more natural and deeply embedded. Even someone who has gained insight into no-self can still experience these afflictions, up to a certain level.

When we talk about the teaching on no-self, we're not rejecting the reality of self and others. Even those who have gained insight into no-self experience this distinction between self and others. Based upon that, you will have thoughts, feelings, and so on. A great scholar and practitioner that I know quite well, and who had in fact gained deep insight into *anatta*, or no-self, once told me that when he tried to meditate on death, which we refer to as meditation on the gross level of impermanence, it really gave him so much stress.

Margaret Kemeny: Now His Holiness is using the word "stress," right?

Alan Wallace: The word that His Holiness actually used, which was translated as "stress," refers to energy in the heart coming out of balance. That needs a little bit of commentary as it taps into traditional Tibetan medicine, which is rooted in ayurveda. Traditional Tibetan medicine speaks of three humors: wind, bile, and phlegm. From a Western medical perspective, they sound completely metaphysical. From the perspective of Tibetan medicine, they're not metaphysical at all, but are immediate contents of experience. They're directly diagnosed by means of pulse and urine analysis.

There are various types of these humors or energies that can be distinguished from a first-person perspective and by highly trained doctors. A particular type of energy within the body is very closely related to the heart. It's actually at the center of the chest but relates to the physical heart as well. Great stress, whether imposed externally by trauma or internally by applying too much mental effort—for example, studying too hard or meditating on something that creates existential angst—can give rise to an imbalance in this energy of the heart. This then manifests as anxiety, depression, being on edge, irritability, insomnia, or loss of appetite. In other words, stress.

Esther Sternberg: So we're really talking about the same thing, but we're using some different terminology.

HH Dalai Lama: That's right. Everybody has the same experience, whether Buddhist or non-Buddhist, whether Christian or nonbelievers. This human body has the same experience.

Esther Sternberg: Another area where we all have the same experience is compassion, and the goal really is for us all to become more compassionate human beings. We keep bringing the topic back to this and asking how cultivating compassion can help health, even if that kind of extrapolation is not part of the Buddhist tradition. I'd like to ask whether a healer, by learning to meditate in this way, can gain compassion and therefore be more able to help those who are ill. At the same time, can compassion be a buffer to stressful events that occur in the brain?

HH Dalai Lama: That's very true. Some of my friends believe that moral ethics must be based on some kind of religious faith, but the Buddhist viewpoint, broadly speaking, is a kind of humanism. The starting point of Buddhism is really the nature of reality and the fact of one's existence, the human condition. Therefore, the Buddhist viewpoint emphasizes affection, compassion, the sense of care, and the sense of concern. Human beings are mammals whose survival is entirely dependent on others' care at the beginning of life, and this is true of many other animals to some extent. Because of that nature, we tend to mentally conflate these elements of care and concern, and we call that affection. Without that, how could we survive? It has nothing to do with religion.

So now we try to sustain that potential. We human beings have the intelligence to recognize that affection and compassion are useful, and we have the ability to sustain them. Other animals have similar mental elements that bind them together at the beginning, when there is a need. When the time arrives that this is not necessary for each others' care, then that affection is no longer there. But human beings, because of our intelligence, can sustain and even increase it. I think Buddhist concepts based on human nature may therefore be easier for nonbelievers to accept.

165

Given that the starting point of Buddhism is really the fact of reality and the existence of the human condition, much of its spiritual approach is really aimed at dealing with the problems of that fact of existence. From the Buddhist point of view, morality or ethics do not necessarily require religious faith as a foundation. Perhaps that makes aspects of Buddhist contemplative practice suitable for adaptation into some health domains.

Esther Sternberg: I thank you for those words because I think ultimately the goal of clinical medicine and the goal of healers is to be compassionate to their patients. We talked briefly yesterday about the placebo effect. The compassionate interaction between doctor and patient has a very powerful effect which perhaps we've lost sight of in some of our modern medical approaches. We need the grounding in science and the technology, where we've made so many advances, but we cannot forget that compassion.

HH Dalai Lama: There is recognition of that even in modern medicine. In Jon Kabat-Zinn's earlier presentation, he made reference to the Hippocratic oath, which is implicit recognition of that grounding in compassion.

Esther Sternberg: I would like to ask Joan Halifax to comment, as this is her area of expertise. She is founder, abbot, and head teacher at the Upaya Zen Center in Santa Fe, New Mexico, and she works with dying patients. Joan, I would like you to comment on your applications of this compassionate approach to preventing stress and easing the dying process.

Joan Halifax: I think that coming to terms with the truth of our mortality as human beings is an essential aspect of our approach as clinicians. The truth of indeterminacy, groundlessness, and impermanence is something that we need to contemplate deeply. But in addition to this, the training of clinicians needs to include a view of health that is not related to just the mind or the body, but also to spirituality, the social realm, and the environment.

Another important aspect has to do with the mental training of clinicians in the areas of attentional balance, emotional balance, metacognition, resilience, and wholesome mental qualities such as empathy, compassion, equanimity, and altruism. These mental qualities, when cultivated and developed, make it possible for clinicians to perform their duties in a more skillful way and can prevent pathologies such as burnout, secondary trauma, moral distress, and horizontal as well as vertical hostility—all challenges that clinicians may face in caring for others or working in medical institutions. One of the essential questions we have to look at is how to educate clinicians in attentional and emotional balance. Meditation is one avenue that can lead to the prevention of suffering, and education in the relevance of empathy, compassion, equanimity, and altruism in clinical medicine is important for clinicians in their interactions with their patients, and as well as for their own mental well-being and maturation.

HH Dalai Lama: The recognition and acceptance of one's mortality is really very crucial. Acceptance that death is inevitable and a part of life makes it much easier for a person when it actually comes. When death comes suddenly for someone who is totally unthinking, that creates much more mental disturbance. On the other hand, if one thinks too much about death, like the Tibetan monk I mentioned earlier, and it leads to stress, that's an unnecessary extreme too.

Joan Halifax: It might depend on how old one is.

HH Dalai Lama: Sometimes I think modern scientists approach a particular area with pinpoint focus, trying to find some absolute, independent answer. That's impossible! Even looking further and further into the smallest of particles, their very existence depends on other particles and is momentarily changing. You can't find something absolute and permanent. That's true even of matter or gross energy, and mind is more subtle. It is very difficult to understand phenomena, particularly mental phenomena, in an isolated context without looking at their relationship to many other factors. One really needs to have a more comprehensive or integrated view, rather than trying to find an absolute location.

Esther Sternberg: I'm so glad you said that, because one of the goals we now have in academic medicine is to try to find a comprehensive, integrative approach—not only an integration between different disciplines, such as we've talked about between neuroscience, psychiatry, psychology, immunology, and cardiology, but an integration of the whole self, of the individual within the larger world. The individual and the larger world are not mutually exclusive. They are one integrated whole.

HH Dalai Lama: Even to experience a mental event, there needs to be a physical basis of some kind. So they are interrelated.

Esther Sternberg: As scientists, we can delve into the minutiae as long as we maintain our compassion, our joy, and our thrill at discovery, which we all have. I think we're all spiritual at heart, and we can combine both worldviews.

Jan Chozen Bays, you commented earlier that you have been involved with treating victims of child abuse and post-traumatic stress disorder. I wonder if you can comment on how meditation and compassion help in those very painful situations.

Jan Chozen Bays: When we're working with illness and human suffering on a daily basis, we need an antidote for that ourselves, and it has to be a spiritual antidote, a spiritual medicine. For example, meditation on a daily basis helps to clear the heart and the mind. Working with child abuse and hearing terrible stories of suffering, I have to meditate every day so that I can clear my heart and my mind to see the next family the next day. It's an absolute necessity. I also need to understand that the parent I'm talking to, who abused a child, now injured or dead, probably was an abused child himself or herself. The cycle of samsara will continue. If I can see those parents as abused children who never received any spiritual tools to help them out of their own suffering, then my heart can stay open to them.

Even if you only have ten minutes to see a patient and to be completely present with that one person, it helps to then clear the heart and mind for two seconds before you move to the next patient. So it becomes an every-few-minutes practice, not something extraordinary that we do on a retreat, twice a year, but something that we have to be doing continuously.

The awareness of our own emptiness is also important. When a family gets angry at me, which happens often, if I can perceive myself as transparent or empty, then what comes toward me can go through me and out the door. I'm not perfect at it, but it's a wonderful way to help work with something.

HH Dalai Lama: Very good.

Jan Chozen Bays: I wanted to ask Your Holiness a question. I have two lives, my medical life and my life in Zen teaching and practice. My medical mind gets very skeptical when someone claims that a medicine can cure everything from A to Z. It sounds like someone selling snake oil. We've been hearing in the last few days that mindfulness-based stress reduction can cure everything from asthma to heart disease to psoriasis. The medical part of me is a little skeptical that this is too simplistic, and that as we unfold this further, it will not be so simple. But the part of me that is a Zen teacher and practitioner sees that when people begin to practice, it's as if they have taken a vitamin, something essential to their health. It could be that meditation practice supplies something as absolutely essential as sleep, or food, or being loved. So I wonder what Your Holiness thinks about this.

HH Dalai Lama: In the Buddhist texts, there are references to arahants who have gained total liberation from the cycle of existence. These are masters who have reached a very high spiritual level, having perfected the four foundations of mindfulness a long time before. But still they are susceptible to illness, old age, and death. So I think it's going too far when some spiritual masters claim that if you practice their meditation, then everything will be all right! The problems of the mind are very complex, so the antidote also must be comprehensive. Mindfulness is just one part of that. It's not that easy.

Joan Halifax: His Holiness is talking about something really essential, which is not disavowing the ethical element, or the experience of deep inquiry, in addition to meditation practice.

Esther Sternberg: This conversation has raised some very interesting similarities and differences between the Buddhist worldview, clinical medicine, and science. By definition, in science we must be objective, as you outlined beautifully in your most recent book, *The Universe in a Single Atom: The Convergence of Science and Spirituality.*[97] We must break down the problem to its smallest parts in order to understand it.

HH Dalai Lama: That's right.

Esther Sternberg: In clinical medicine we have to take a wider view. I think there is more of a synergy between Buddhism and clinical medicine than there is between Buddhism and science. That doesn't mean that we can't blend the science with the clinical medicine, and it doesn't mean, as you have pointed out so eloquently in your book, that we shouldn't also blend the science with different worldviews. In fact, in this day of globalized ideas, blending all these traditions with what we know through modern science is essential to a fuller understanding of the world.

Richard Davidson: Your Holiness, a question about mind/body interaction was raised in various ways by members of the audience as well as by the speakers when we discussed this at lunch. Many meditation practices involve focusing attention on particular parts of the body, and other meditation practices involve spontaneous attention to bodily processes. In the Buddhist understanding, when we place our awareness in a particular part of the body, is that part of the body in any way changed?

HH Dalai Lama: It depends upon the degree of mastery the individual has in the application of sustained attention. If the individual has a very high level of stability, or focused attention, there is an understanding that there could be a change on the physical level as well. For example, in some of the texts that talk about the Buddhist theory of energy, there are discussions about how it can have a physiological effect if an advanced meditator who has gained mastery over this application of sustained attention can maintain that focus of energy on a particular point of the body for over four hours, unwaveringly. One or two hours of meditation on a particular area won't work.

Richard Davidson: We need many more years of practice.

HH Dalai Lama: For me, analytical meditation is more useful, just analyzing the pain. For example, when you experience a trauma, that experience has already occurred.

I mentioned at the beginning that many problems are essentially due to ignorance. Ignorance brings with it an unrealistic attitude. And unrealistic attitude brings a lot of mental problems. Accept reality, and approach it more realistically. If something can be done, there's no need to worry. If it cannot be done, there's no use worrying. Finished.

One source of problems is grasping at some sort of enduring permanence. Another source of problems is extreme self-centeredness. For each of these mental ailments, we need different approaches, different antidotes to transform and shape the mind. That's my view. To realize intelligence more effectively, I prefer a sound sleep more than meditation!

Esther Sternberg: I think perhaps, with that, you deserve a sound sleep!

HH Dalai Lama: Thank you!

SESSION 5

INTEGRATION AND FINAL REFLECTIONS

In this session, moderated by Bennett Shapiro, presenters reflect on the major themes elucidated during the presentations and dialogues in earlier sessions. The first presentation focuses on the roles that meditation and, more broadly, integrative approaches might play in the evolution of health care. The second presentation offers a sweeping view of the nature of mind and self, the inherent limitations in human perceptions of these constructs, and the immense potential that lies in bridging the contemplative and scientific traditions.

Bennett Shapiro: This has been a most engaging and provocative meeting for all of us. I'd like to offer some thoughts on the past few days, but I have to give a disclaimer. I am not a neuroscientist, nor am I a psychologist. I am a physician who pursued a career in biochemistry and molecular biology. For many years I was a professor of biochemistry, and then entered the area of drug discovery in an attempt to find breakthrough medicines for serious diseases. I've been doing that for the past fifteen years, partly in a large pharmaceutical company and partly in biotechnology.

So I've been working at the center of reductionist biology, which has had such a powerful effect in transforming the way we look at the living process. When I began my career, I could never have imagined that we would have the insights we have today about the nature of life and the interconnectedness of all living organisms. These insights have emerged from the deep analytic approach taken during the past half century or more, when the techniques and ideas of physics and chemistry were applied to biology. Mixing such powerful ideas and technologies has truly led to a revolution in our understanding of the nature of life and our ability to discover novel therapies to help relieve suffering.

No field has benefited as much from the introduction of physics and chemistry to biology as neuroscience. In fact the whole field has been transformed. We now understand a great deal about how nerve cells work, how they're integrated, and the chemistry of their activities. The progress has been unimaginable. Yet we have not made similar progress in understanding the mind. Although we have deep understanding about the nature of the brain, our progress in understanding the mind has been very slow. Western attempts at studying the mind were derailed for several reasons, one of which was the enormous impetus of behaviorism. When it became clear at the end of the nineteenth century that people could not report internal states very well, psychology shifted considerably to looking at external behavior as an index of what occurs inside. Indeed, for the first half of the twentieth century, people ignored internal mental states almost completely. A few theories of mind emerged, including those of Freud and others, but the mainstream of psychological research dealt with behaviors, both in animals and in people. Only in the last twenty or twenty-five years has it been legitimate to talk about consciousness, which is at the core of our very being.

The question is, How do we make progress in this area? We need to apply powerful technology and novel insights. Most of the ways that we have illuminated specific issues about the human mind have involved looking at people with strokes or other brain injuries, determining what was lost, and inferring from their thinking and behavior what these parts of the brain do. Or we have looked at undergraduate students and asked them many questions in psychology laboratories all around the world. We've done any number of experiments with this cadre of young people in psychology departments to try to infer the potential of the human mind.

When I think back on my time as an undergraduate, I was not achieving the highest potential of the human mind. I don't believe that many of us would consider our minds at the end of our teenage years to be the acme of human potential. One could ask a reasonable question: Where can we turn to understand the potential of the mind? We all have agreed that we need to somehow improve what our minds, these powerful tools, are doing to our health and our planet. Where do we find ways to understand what the potential of the human mind really is?

To me, it's not unreasonable to look to people who have enormous expertise in this area. It seems the most reasonable thing to do from a scientific point of view, much as we would make those decisions in any other area we investigate. As a reductionist molecular scientist, it seems to me most reasonable to look at a culture that has spent thousands of years developing mental insight, as in the contemplative aspects of Buddhism or Christianity, and to seek the perspective of those who have spent tens of thousands of hours in meditation and have used rigorous technologies of their own to investigate the mind in many different ways that they can describe to each other, and that they say are reproducible. These are people who have the equivalent experience of four or five PhDs, the equivalent of medical training with many years of specialty training and practice. If you were going to have cardiac surgery, it is unlikely that any of you would turn to an undergraduate student. I'm not speaking against undergraduate students, having been there myself and having parented teenagers, but I think one has to approach this realistically. If we are asking about something as serious as the potential of the human mind, it seems to me only reasonable that we would go to people who have studied it.

So it's no surprise that the wise leadership of the Society for Neuroscience would have invited His Holiness to come and speak to their national meeting here in Washington, DC, just the other day. Where else would you turn, logically, if you're really interested in challenging neuroscience to take a serious look at the mind? It seems obvious on the face of it that this makes perfect, incontrovertible sense. Contemplatives have many years of experience investigating the mind inwardly. Why not ask them? Additionally, if we had a clearer idea of the mind and its interactions, coupled with everything we know about physical reality, we could help heal some of the challenges that medicine is facing, as well as other painful aspects of our society.

The opportunity is just enormous. It is the same opportunity that existed in the 1930s, when physicists and chemists started getting more serious about biology. All of human progress that is based on technological innovation has very much depended on the introduction of new ideas into established areas. That's how you make quantum leaps in understanding. In this case, we have an opportunity, thanks to His Holiness, the Mind and Life Institute, and others who are interested in this area, to look at problems that we've engaged with the tools of Western science in a completely distinct way—to ask questions, collaborate, and gain insights in how to address these problems. This dialogue can have the same kind of profoundly transformative impact on what we're doing over the next fifty years that physics and chemistry had on our understanding of biology. We're asking for two major intellectual disciplines to interface with each other, and we don't know where it will lead.

In addition to this wonderful opportunity, there also are great challenges. The first is an attitudinal challenge, the tendency of some physicians to reject a mechanistic link between the mind and physical illness. Although there is a legitimate and important journal today called *Psychosomatic Medicine*, when I was training as a doctor, a psychosomatic illness was seen by many doctors as not really illness at all, but some type of intellectual dishonesty on the part of the patient. That's a very strange idea for a medical practitioner.

There are attitudes that must be changed and it will take time to change them. What can a Tibetan monk possibly tell neuroscientists? A handful of people have raised that question in reference to His Holiness speaking at the meeting of the Society for Neuroscience. Clearly those attitudes exist whenever any revolutionary idea arises. There are always people who are much more comfortable not even thinking about the potential for a revolution in our understanding.

There are operational challenges as well. I'm an outsider to much of what's going on here, but I do know a fair amount about drug discovery. Let me tell you what we go through when we're trying to discover a breakthrough medicine, to prove that it actually works in people—because it's very important to be sure that any new therapy you impose is effective and safe. When we do complex clinical trials, we use placebos that are exactly matched in shape, form, taste, and all visible properties to the drug that we're testing. We do that because the placebo effect, which is a surrogate for the power of the mind, can be enormous in these clinical trials. On trials of pain medication, it could be very large. On trials of depression medication, it is often so large that the drug itself is no different than placebo. Even in trials on blood pressure, swelling of the joints in arthritis, or obstruction to urine flow, there is a substantial placebo effect. In many of these trials, if the total effect size is 50 percent, the placebo effect alone might be 20 or 30 percent. We also use completely randomized populations to make sure that the backgrounds and characteristics of the people getting the drug are identical to those of the people getting the placebo. We use a triple-blinded technique in clinical trials: the patient doesn't know whether she or he is getting the drug, the doctor doesn't know, and the person calculating the coded data doesn't know. There's no possibility for bias. Although it's very artificial, we view this as the highest standard.

When we look at how difficult it would be to apply this standard to the study of meditation, we can understand the challenges that our colleagues face in the experiments they have introduced to you. Clearly it's very hard to find an identical placebo group. A waiting period may distinguish the treated and not treated groups, but it's very hard to randomize because many people who volunteer for these trials are enthusiastic about meditation or have meditated in the past. We're still in the stage of developing techniques for reporting internal states, and these need to be optimized. We're exploring the use of biomarkers and imaging technology to help guide thinking in this area.

It's clear that these are very early investigations. It is unrealistic to assume that all of the technology has been perfected in the first years of exploring this area. But the courage and enthusiasm of the people involved indicate that there is enormous potential here. We've heard in this meeting many indications of how powerful the mind can be when explored carefully in different settings. We've talked about how experienced contemplatives are adding value to such investigations, and we've begun to see in early experiments from Richard Davidson's and others' laboratories that there is an even greater potential within the human mind, brain, and body than earlier studies had suggested.

The third issue that we have to consider is ethical. Today, I think all of us believe that mental training is an extremely powerful technology—I certainly do. You can see the damage that occurs when the mind goes in the wrong direction. There is no more powerful weapon than the human mind. And so we are really fortunate, and we should pause and think about the fact that these disciplines involving tens of thousands of hours of meditation practice were developed in the context of religious traditions grounded in moral motivation. That is not a problem; that is a blessing. One could imagine these technologies being inappropriately used. I should just remind you that the whole project of mindfulness-based stress reduction is grounded in this same ethical base, because the people developing it recognized how important that part of the process was. But it's possible that one could develop similar technologies of mind training with no concern for ethics—an extremely unattractive possibility.

In the early stages of a field like this, it's useful to consider what problems might emerge from refining the approach to ensure that, as we move ahead, we're committed not only to the highest standards of scientific excellence, but also the same high standards of ethics and morality that have supported the development of these meditative technologies over thousands of years. That's our responsibility as well as our challenge as we proceed.

I believe that we are witnessing the birth of an approach that has the opportunity to transform not only medicine and health but much of human suffering in an extremely powerful way, if we continue to develop it wisely. And so I have to offer my deepest personal gratitude to His Holiness, to the memory of Francisco Varela, and to Adam Engle and our other colleagues who have been associated with the Mind and Life Institute for so many years, for initiating this dialogue that has so much potential to relieve human suffering.

This morning, we'll hear the perspectives of two extremely distinguished individuals. Our first speaker is Ralph Snyderman, who is one of America's most eminent medical leaders and educators. A physician and a scientist, he has been head of the Duke University Health System for many years. He continues to be actively engaged in all aspects of health care. We're delighted, Ralph, that you can spend some time with us.

RALPH SNYDERMAN *Meditation and the Future of Health Care*

Medicine is moving inexorably toward a more integrative perspective on many fronts, as emerging technologies and expanded epistemologies are incorporated into how medicine is practiced. This presentation considers the ways in which what has been discussed thus far in Mind and Life XIII, from both the clinical and the basic science perspectives, might contribute to this ongoing development in medical care, medical education, and medical research. It also addresses the potential this integrated approach offers for creating more rational institutional approaches to health and well-being, as well as elucidating a larger role for engaged participation on the part of individuals in furthering their own health.

Your Holiness, it is truly a pleasure and an important moment for all of us, assembled here from different paths, to be with you. Every one of those paths is distinct and important. Nonetheless, we're all together here in this room at this moment wanting to improve the human condition, to minimize human suffering, and to liberate people from distress.

My particular path has been as a physician. My calling has been as a healer of human suffering of the body. What I have found through my forty years of being a physician, with the full power of Western science and technology, conducting research in many fields of medicine, is that the power and tools of science and technology, while vast, are insufficient of themselves to minimize suffering and enhance well-being.

For that reason, I and many of my colleagues, and I suspect many of the people in this room, are coming to you and your colleagues to learn of the wisdom gained from over two thousand years of introspective contemplation, to determine what could be applied to improve the human condition. The Mind and Life meetings, for which we are so grateful, indicate that you also feel that the tremendous power and learning the Buddhist tradition has achieved can benefit from a deeper understanding of science. This is natural. What can we learn from each other, and how can these two approaches strengthen one another?

This particular Mind and Life meeting continues a journey down a pathway that has developed over the course of thirteen meetings. The point of this meeting is to determine what we have learned and what we can learn about mental training and mindfulness, to improve our understanding of the importance of the brain in health—not only mental health, but physical health. Where can we go from here? Can we use the tools and understanding we have gathered here to go forward and make things better for the future?

During this meeting, we have learned a great deal by discussing findings from two radically different approaches to understanding the mind. We have learned that focusing and training the mind can have a very powerful impact on the structure and function of the brain, and that if we use this knowledge, perhaps we can do things that will improve the human condition. We have learned that mental training and meditation can change the structure of the brain. They can alter the neural networks of the brain through plasticity, with changes such as modifications of neural connections. Mental training can enhance the activity of portions of the brain that seem to be related to compassion. It can minimize the power of the portion of the brain that controls fear, anxiety, and anger. That's a powerful message.

We have also learned a bit about the very mysterious ways the brain works, with the information that's processed during thinking being totally distributive, with no central locus of control. We have learned that mental training can coordinate the oscillations of the functions of the different parts of the brain. We have learned that destructive emotions, such as anger, fear, shock, and grief, as well as stress of various kinds, all cause changes not only in the mind but in the body and brain. We have learned that mental training can change this. The Buddhists have known this for over two thousand years, but the data have now shown that mental training can actually change physiological processes to the benefit of the individual.

Stress can cause changes in blood flow to the heart. It can cause heart attacks and ulcers, can decrease resistance to many other diseases, and can cause clinical depression, which is one of the most painful mental sufferings. Clinical depression is associated with abnormalities in the functioning of the brain, and mental training, to a degree, can improve those functions that help decrease clinical depression. It is very powerful. It's not a cure, but it is a supplement to dealing with a very painful human condition.

Through the work of Dr. Jon Kabat-Zinn on mindfulness-based stress reduction and the work of his colleagues who developed mindfulness-based cognitive therapy, we have learned that meditation training can be beneficial for large numbers of ordinary people who are neither Buddhists nor monastics. Mindfulness training can alleviate the pain and suffering of many people. The application of such meditative approaches to the trajectory of chronic disease is now a matter of intense interest and an important area of discussion.

The path I have taken as a physician has shown me that pure science and technology can lead in a direction that is to some degree a dead end. By itself, science doesn't solve all clinical problems, and in some ways it can create even more problems.

The practice of medicine in the Western world has evolved dramatically over the last one hundred years. Hippocrates, in about 500 BC, was the first to establish a code of ethics in Western medicine. He was also responsible for separating medicine from mythology and putting medicine on an objective basis wherein we learn from what we observe. In the 1600s, it was shown that the heart, which had been thought to be an almost mystical object, was truly a muscle that pumped blood. This differentiated the organ in the human body from more spiritual ideas associated with the heart.

In 1847, Dr. Ignaz Semmelweis, a key figure in the history of medicine who hasn't received sufficient recognition for his enormous contributions, was working in Austria in the best hospital in the Western world at that time. They were faced with a tremendous problem: Women who gave birth frequently died in a few days from severe fever associated with inflammation and pus in the female reproductive tract. This was called puerperal sepsis, or childbed fever. Dr. Semmelweis noticed that the incidence of childbed fever was very high in women whose babies were delivered by doctors. If the women had babies delivered by midwives, the incidence was much lower. At that time, doctors learned by performing autopsies in the morning on women who had died the day before of childbed fever. They didn't wash their hands because there was no concept of germs. They would then deliver the babies of women who, in turn, would develop childbed fever. Dr. Semmelweis realized the hands of the doctors going from the women who had died to the normal women must be transmitting something that caused the disease. You'd think doctors would have said, "Hallelujah! It's wonderful that we finally understand!" However, they rejected the idea. Dr. Semmelweis was considered crazy and cast as a villain. Doctors at that time believed that childbed fever was caused by a miasma in the atmosphere or a problem with the humors, such as bile and phlegm. This was one instance in which the medical profession totally rejected something that they were not ready to accept because, in part, there was no framework for understanding the new concept.

It was only later, when the causative agents were clearly identified through the work of Robert Koch, Louis Pasteur, and Joseph Lister, that it became accepted that germs cause disease. Koch discovered that a microscopic agent was the cause of tuberculosis and showed this with total certainty, leading to a revolution in medicine. All of a sudden, science and technology seemed to hold tremendous power, once it was understood that so many diseases were caused by infectious agents, and powerful new technologies could be developed to treat them with great specificity. This naturally gave rise to a "find it and fix it" culture.

Over the last one hundred years, medical science has given rise to many wonderful things. However, it is now very heavily focused on disease. We spend almost no time on health. We make an assumption that for every disease, there is a defect that we need to find and fix. We don't deal with people throughout their lives, but only when they're sick. In the United States, we have become accustomed to assuming that one's health is managed by one's doctor, and that individuals have little responsibility or control over their health.

Where does this leave us? On the one hand, life expectancy in 1900 was forty years. Today it's eighty years. We have doubled life expectancy in a hundred years. That's almost miraculous. On the other hand, in 1900 the most likely cause of death for a young man between the ages of fifteen and twenty-five would have been infection. Today, it's murder, suicide, drug abuse, or violent accidents. We have made tremendous progress, but some of the consequences of our progress are absolutely terrifying. In addition, we have a tremendous accumulation of chronic diseases, many of which are fostered by people's own behavior.

One of the problems with Western medicine is that it tends to make a reductionist assumption that for every disease, there is a single causative factor that we need to find and fix. We now are learning that there are often multiple factors, rather than a single reductionist cause of disease. People are born with a baseline risk, and then environmental factors impinge on that risk over time. There is a tremendous difference in susceptibility to different diseases, yet we often have a lot of control over environmental factors that contribute to disease progression.

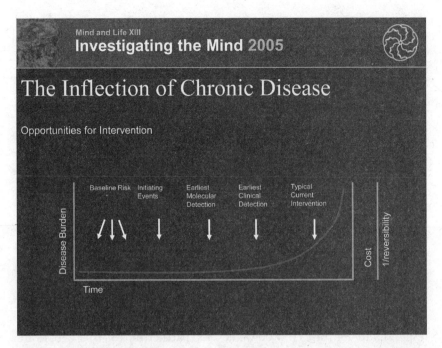

Figure 11. Disease develops as a consequence of inherited susceptibility (genetic inheritance) and exposure to environmental factors, including lifestyle. For a long portion of their development, many diseases are not clinically apparent, although in many cases they could be detected with appropriate attention and diagnostics. Once signs and symptoms develop, it is generally late in the disease development process, and the degree of reversibility is reduced and the cost of treatment is increased compared to interventions at an earlier time.

Think of a chronic disease such as tuberculosis. People are born with a baseline risk, and they then may get exposed over a period of time. If everybody in this auditorium was exposed to the bacterium that causes tuberculosis, a small number of people would have a very serious problem and probably would not survive. Many people would have almost no effects whatsoever. In the middle, there would be a broad range of responses to the same bacterium. In other words, even though the tuberculosis bacterium causes a disease, its effects are dependent on far more complex factors related to an individual's resistance or susceptibility.

It's the same with virtually any disease. Diseases develop over time as a consequence of an individual's inherited susceptibility, or genetics, and what he or she has been exposed to or has experienced throughout life. In the United States today, the health care system tends to focus on disease very late in its development. Over time, the ability to cure the disease or minimize its effects decreases, and the cost of treating it increases. However, we are now entering an era when we will be able to predict disease much earlier. With personalized health care, the focus is on prevention and disease minimization. This requires individuals to understand their health risks and engage in behaviors and, when appropriate, therapies that minimize the risks of disease progression. I believe that in our lifetimes we will have the capability to determine an individual's risk for problems long before they occur. This will give individuals more opportunity, responsibility, and control over their own health.

The problem is, at least in the United States, people don't seem to want to assume that responsibility. In the new world of health care, where we can predict and prevent disease, the role of the individual becomes more powerful. This is why we need to come to you, Your Holiness, for advice. As the role of the individual becomes more important, how do we encourage people to be aware that health is a value and that they have responsibility for this? How do we develop partnerships so that people are willing to take it upon themselves to develop and meet goals and modify their behavior appropriately? We believe that stress reduction, a quiet mind, a forgiving mind, and a compassionate mind are essential to promoting health. As we think about meditation promoting ethical values, in my very naive way I wonder if how one treats one's body, and how one might stop abusing one's body, would be part of embodying ethical values.

Let me summarize what we have learned in this meeting and see if it has relevance for health care, at least from my perspective. We have learned that meditation, or mental training, is capable of modifying neural networks and coordinating regional brain oscillations. Meditation is a very powerful tool. It modulates neuroendocrine functions—hormones that have powerful effects on virtually every system in the body. We have learned that meditation enhances awareness and engagement and potentially enhances wellness through improving the immune system. It may actually limit disease. From Jon Kabat-Zinn's presentation on psoriasis and from other presentations about the impact of the mind on pathology, we know that, at a minimum, the mind can help limit suffering from pain. We heard the story of being shot by an arrow once but having the pain twice.

We have the pain from the physical event, but using the powerful tools of meditation and mindfulness can help us avoid having the mind distort the pain and make it much worse than it is—the second arrow.

Your Holiness, a question I have for you and your colleagues is, Are there aspects of meditative practices that enhance compassion, which could turn that compassion inward to ourselves and our own bodies? Can we use aspects of mental training to engage people in their own health during their lifetimes?

Let me end by saying that, for me, this is one of the most wonderful moments of my life, being here with you, and I'm grateful to everybody here for allowing me to participate in this collective inquiry.

Bennett Shapiro: Our next speaker is Wolf Singer, who also presented in session 2. Wolf is a distinguished neuroscientist who has given us profound insights into the nature of relationships within the brain. He will now offer his perspective on what has been presented during this dialogue.

WOLF SINGER *Some Reflections on the Evolution and Nature of Mind and Self, and Their Implications for Humanity*

Within the cross-fertilization of approaches that this meeting represents, a number of epistemological conundrums arise, both on the science side and on the contemplative side. These final reflections address a range of themes and concerns that emerged during the dialogue, including the strong habit of reifying a self-identity that cannot be found, and the apparent and humbling limits of our capacity as a species for knowing, particularly when viewed through the lenses of evolutionary biology, philosophy, or neuroscience. How does a group of neurons or the whole brain or an individual or a society know when it has arrived at a coherent or optimal solution to a problem? How do we value the deep beauty of what science offers at its best, as well as keep in mind its limitations and that it is one way of knowing among others that also have profound validity? How do we maintain and implement the best of what the contemplative traditions provide us? How do we deal wisely and compassionately with our own helplessness, with uncertainty and with the limitations of our understanding? How can the richness of the present dialogue, and the confluence of these different ways of knowing that the sciences and contemplative practices represent, further such inquiries and their translation into effective strategies for investigation and for humane action going forward?

Your Holiness, it is a great honor to be back here with you again, to share these last moments of the conference and to convey some of the ideas that came to my mind while I was listening to the presentations and discussions.

Much of this conference has been based on deep sources of wisdom and knowledge, and therefore I consider it appropriate to begin with a few epistemic considerations. Of course, I shall approach this from a neurobiological perspective because this is the only perspective I'm familiar with. It is important to consider that what we can know or imagine about the world is limited, constrained by the cognitive abilities of our brains. Our brains are the product of an evolutionary process, so they have been arranged through trial and error and adapted to our world. This suggests that the human brain probably has not been optimized to discover the absolute truth behind phenomena, in Kant's sense. Rather, it predicts that our brains have implemented pragmatic strategies of survival to keep the organisms that possess them alive in a world that is full of uncertainties and dangers.

To fulfill this function, brains have adapted to a world defined at the level of centimeters and meters, because this is the scale at which we exist as organisms. This is the world of classical physics, where the coordinates of time and space are fixed and unchanging, not relative. This is probably why it is so difficult for us to imagine or understand intuitively processes at the quantum level and at cosmic dimensions. We have no intuition for these processes because we did not need to understand them in order to survive. And probably for the same reason, we have poor intuition for the dynamics of very complex, nonlinear systems. What our brains are driven to do is make models of the world to derive predictions for further action. It's better to know when the tiger is coming than to be surprised and get eaten.

However, it is only possible to make predictions in a linear process where causality is a simple principle. Therefore we seem to have an innate inclination to assume that the world is linear and simple, whereas, of course, it is not. This preconception of how the world is organized worked well when our brains were being shaped in evolution, when we were still monkeys. This simpleminded assumption is probably what made us also assume that somewhere in the brain we must have this mover or self that we talked about.

We assume as well that the brain works like a linear machine, following the same material processes of classical physics as do clocks and simple machines. Yet we know that linear systems are not creative or intentional. They cannot take initiative, and they are not capable of producing surprises. However, we experience ourselves as creative, intentional, open toward the future, indeterminate, and free, and we observe others as being the same. Since we assume linearity, we think there must be something in the brain that makes all those wonderful things happen. This is probably why we postulate this mover to whom we attribute the mysterious properties of an immaterial self.

The scientific approach has now shown that the brain is not a simple, linear machine, but a highly complex, self-organizing system with very nonlinear dynamics that operates far from equilibrium. Such systems have all the properties that we usually attribute to the immaterial mind; for example, they can be creative and open to the future. A particularly important property of such systems is that they can support the emergence of new qualities, qualities that cannot be deduced from the properties of the components—qualities such as intentionality or consciousness or morality. It is an interesting puzzle that this system, with all its intuitions and conceptions and wonderful functions, has so little understanding of how it actually works. We don't feel the mind at work. It is a fantastic internal misappraisal.

This situation, particularly in the Western world, has led to a conceptual dichotomy or dualism between the world in its material manifestation, which is the fully predictable world of classical physics, and, on the other side, a mental world, which is immaterial, devoid of any constraints, and fully indeterminate. This view, as we now know, is in conflict with Western science and much less in conflict with Eastern intuition, for interesting reasons.

This view of the world is, in part, responsible for two very characteristic attitudes of Western civilization. One is our strong emphasis on the self as the essence of everything: the autonomous, free, and hence fully responsible mover who is more or less almighty. A second attitude that is very pronounced in the West because of this conceptual dichotomy is that we, the conscious self, think that we can fully control and direct this stupid, simple, mechanical world.

It is fascinating to me that other cultures, especially Eastern cultures, have developed a very different intuition about the position of the self in the world, and about the organization of the world, an intuition that is apparently much less in conflict with modern science than our traditional Cartesian Western intuition. I don't know why this strange bifurcation in cultural development occurred. This would be an interesting topic of study.

A couple of years ago, I asked a Chinese colleague, "How is it that your cultural development has been so conservative? Why has there not been all the turmoil as in the West, moving from classic philosophy and architecture to Gothic and Baroque, and then the Enlightenment, and so on?" His simple answer was, "Because we had the right intuition from the beginning, so no further search was required." He added that maybe this was also the reason why they did not have to develop the kind of analytical sciences that we have here in the West, but directed their search toward the inner world.

Here then is a very curious bifurcation of cultural evolution that led to widely divergent views of the human condition, and then as a consequence to radically different concepts of the self and two very different strategies for exploring the world. On one side are the spiritual techniques of self-exploration through meditation, a method that is entirely dominated by the first-person perspective. We in the West, with our scientific approach, opted for the third-person perspective, analyzing things from the outside.

This raises an interesting question: How do we know which view is the "right" one? If this is not a silly question to begin with, it may nonetheless be an ill-posed question because it boils down to the conclusion that we have two sources of knowledge: one relying on intuition, self-exploration, and the first-person perspective, and the other, Western science, relying on observation, analytical formulas, and description.

Ultimately, the real question is, How does the brain, which performs all this cognition, know when it is right? This is equally important for scientists and for meditators. How does the brain know when it has reached a correct state? When the search process converges on a result, how do we know how reliable this result is? In essence, there are only complex patterns of activity, so how does it distinguish a pattern that is nonsense or a pattern that is generated while it is looking for a solution from a pattern that *is* a good solution? We have no answer to this interesting question. It should be a whole field of research. But one can speculate, and while I was listening to what the practitioners of meditation said here, it occurred to me that maybe good solutions, or what we might call result states or solution states, are very coherent states where a sufficiently large number of neurons, distributed over a significantly wide area of the brain, get into coherent, stable activation patterns that are maintained for a sufficiently long period of time that they convince the rest of the brain that this is the best result in the moment.

We don't know, but it could be that meditative states tend toward such solutions. What we do know is that the brain has systems for the evaluation of internal states, and when it reaches a result, these systems create pleasant feelings. The aha! or eureka! experience is always associated with a pleasant feeling. We like to find a solution. Meditation might be a strategy that the brain uses to strive toward such pleasant states, where controversies are resolved at the level of both conscious arguments and subconscious competition. There are always many states competing to win, and somehow they have to be reconciled. Maybe meditation is one way to get these many different agents that work in parallel to temporarily make peace.

This leaves us with some interesting questions. The first is, How can a distributed self-organizing system impose on itself a programming strategy that favors the generation of such solution states? How can the system itself make itself get there? I don't know how this is possible. The second interesting question is whether we can be confident that when the system intentionally cultivates awareness of itself, it converges toward good state. Could it also run into a deleterious bifurcation?

Finally, this raises a question alluded to several times during the meeting: whether we need to rely on the wisdom that has been accumulated through trial and error over millennia by the practitioners of Eastern meditation techniques in order to get it right. Of course, when we do this, we should rely on careful supervision, as we would with any other technique. As was said, you wouldn't go to a grad student to get your heart fixed.

However, perhaps there is a different possibility. It could be that evolution has endowed the brain with self-stabilizing mechanisms so that it always safely enters a good state if we leave it in its default mode—if we just decouple it from the disturbing outer world and let it run by itself. Maybe it's done that way. That would be even better.

I would like to conclude with a thought experiment that establishes a link between two complex systems that exist on very different scales—our brains and our societies. They seem to have very similar properties, even though they look quite different. This experiment will make it very clear that it is high time to reconcile science with Western and Eastern intuitions if we want to be able to cope both with the practical and the psychological challenges that we will face in the near future, and are already facing now. The experiment goes as follows: If one asks a neuron in the brain, "What are you doing?" the neuron would say, "I am sitting here comfortably, with many other neurons around me. I'm getting signals from ten thousand others. I do some very simple calculations, and then I send a signal to another ten thousand." This neuron would never tell you that it is part of a machine that generates consciousness, empathy, feelings—nothing like that. It has no concept of responsibility whatsoever.

One gets a similarly restrained answer by asking a member of human society, "What are you doing?" The human being would tell you, "I am embedded in a family and I have children, and I educate. I do this and that . . ." But this answer falls short of the response of someone who could view this whole cultural system from above as the trajectory of the evolution of life on this planet. It is as incomplete with respect to what it means to be integrated in this body of life as is the answer the neuron might give relative to what the brain does. Even though we are the agents who make life on this planet move, cultures evolve, and conditions change, we don't really know the quality of the whole. It's nearly certain that we lack the intelligence to understand the larger conditions, particularly if one considers the evolutionary constraints of our cognitive systems. We were not built to understand these things.

What is certain is that we cannot control the system within which we evolved. Even if we knew more, we would not be able to control its dynamics because it's an evolutionary system. It's nonlinear. Even if we turn screws, thinking we want the system to move in a particular direction, it will go somewhere else. We cannot deliberately steer systems like our economic systems and our social systems. It is impossible in principle. This is what modern science tells us, and I think we are already experiencing this now. All these linear strategies worked well when the world was still simple and our ancestors were jumping around between trees, but it is no longer so.

We are starting to feel that we can no longer control the dynamic processes that we generate, and this gives us a feeling of helplessness and abandonment. It hits Western civilization particularly harshly because of our well-nourished illusion that the almighty self can control everything. I think there's a real danger in the West, and we can see the signs very clearly here in Washington, in particular, of a collective depression because of this collective feeling of helplessness, which in turn engenders the danger of biting our neighbors for relief, as we saw in the experiments with rats described by Robert Sapolsky.

What lessons can we learn from this? Here are a few things I've learned from this meeting, and I'm very grateful for them, though I don't know whether they will translate into normal life tomorrow morning when all the neuroscience competition starts up again. The first message is, let's try to become more humble, given the understanding that there is so much we cannot know. We Westerners should probably reduce the emphasis we put on the almighty self. We will have to learn to befriend and work with the sense of helplessness, because it will not go away. We will have to find peace in ourselves in the present rather than through biting others, if possible. We will have to learn to enjoy openness, to be comfortable with "maybe" and not look for certainties, because we won't be able to attain them. This is particularly important in light of ongoing globalization. We will have to develop what I call "long-distance compassion": the ability to care for those who are remote. That is very difficult for us.

This conference has shown quite clearly that some of those traits can be learned through mental practices, and that we should take advantage of this opportunity. Of course, we should not abandon Western achievements. We should not deconstruct the concept of the responsible self. What we should reduce is the selfish self, the self who finds its only satisfaction in what we call self-realization. We also should not abandon science. On the contrary, we will need science to survive, but we need to give it the place it merits. It is just one of several sources of knowledge.

Conversely, Eastern societies should not sacrifice their achievements for the sake of striving solely toward Western achievements.

Ahead of us lies a difficult responsibility and obligation to select and mutually adopt strategies for coping with life that have evolved independently in different cultures. They should in principle be mergeable and compatible, because they evolved in the same world for the solution of the same problems everywhere.

HH Dalai Lama: Wonderful, wonderful.

SESSION 5 DIALOGUE

In addition to HH Dalai Lama and the presenters, translators, and moderator, panelists for this session include Richard Davidson, Jon Kabat-Zinn, Father Thomas Keating, Matthieu Ricard, and Sharon Salzberg.

Bennett Shapiro: Your Holiness, you spoke yesterday about the concept of the self, and it would be very illuminating if now you could expand upon this issue of the self and its interactions, whether confused, damaging, or helpful, with the rest of being. In Western society we've been damaged so much and yet helped so much by the idea of the individual and the need to integrate the individual in a positive way. I know that the self has been a central aspect of Buddhist thinking, and it would be most interesting to hear your thoughts on some of these ideas.

HH Dalai Lama: Probably humility is the best answer, as Wolf pointed out. I think the human mind has a desire to know everything. The concept of enlightenment comes from that. So that means we accept that our knowledge is, in any case, limited.

Listening to Wolf's wonderful presentation, and particularly the point he made about how it is almost impossible to account for the emergence of mental processes, or their nature, simply on the basis of a linear, materialistic, deterministic account, seems to suggest that what the Buddhists call mental states or consciousness is a kind of energy that results from coherent synchronization in the brain, or whatever the reason may be. Because of that situation, the concept of God also arises, as well as our intuition that there is some kind of controller, or self.

In India, almost three thousand years ago, intelligent people began to investigate where the "I" is located. They had the concept that an independent "I" must exist. Later the Buddha taught that there is no unchanging, permanent self. Rather, the self or "I" is something conceptually imputed on the combination of the body and mind. It is just designated, or conceptually projected, so we cannot find self as a thing with its own entity or its own reality.

This relates to one's philosophical understanding of the nature of reality and what kinds of things exist in the world. One of the things that ancient Indian philosophy, including Buddhist philosophy, postulated is that, aside from physical and mental events, there are phenomena that can only be accepted as constructs of the mind. These are referred to as composite things or mental constructs, and their identity and reality can only be understood in terms of something other than themselves, whether physical or mental events.

In another discussion I asked the scientists whether it is possible on the basis of brain expressions to distinguish between a valid or veridical mental state and a delusional state. This is similar to Wolf's question about the reflexive activity of cognition: How does it know that it's right? In Buddhist epistemology, a distinction is made between sensory experiences on the one hand and mental experiences of thoughts and emotions on the other. For sensory perceptions, the content of that experience is understood to be simply the object perceived. If you have a visual perception of a blue object, for example, there is no reflexive aspect to that experience. From the Buddhist point of view, the reflexivity has to come subsequently and occurs at the mental level of thought: "Yes, I'm seeing a blue object. This is blue." This seems to be quite similar to your intuition that on the individual neuronal level, there is no reflexive quality. Neurons are simply performing whatever function they are doing, whereas the second order of cognition has to occur on a different level. Even in the mental domain, it would be very difficult for individual events of mental experience—say, for example, cognition of a particular state of affairs—to have this second order of reflexive awareness that could verify, "This is truth; this is correct." That validation really has to come from a subsequent experience, or in relation to some other experience.

In Buddhist epistemological texts, particularly those of the middle way or Madhyamaka school, there is the discussion of how a particular cognitive event is determined to be valid. First of all, it must relate to the object, whatever that object may be. Second, that cognition should not be contradicted by other valid experiences that one has had. This suggests that the validation of a mental experience can only occur within the context of other confirming experiences. A third and very specifically Buddhist criterion is that this cognition should not be controverted even by insight into the deeper nature of reality. This may have some connection to the points you raised.

Matthieu Ricard: In former meetings between Alan, Richie, and other friends, we have tried to be more explicit about a definition of well-being that entails a better understanding of reality. The Buddhist notion of sukkha, which is roughly translated as "happiness," refers to an optimally healthy state of mind that suffuses all emotional states and can remain robust and stable through the ups and downs that may come one's way in life. If pleasure and pain, positive or adverse circumstances, are like the different states on the surface of the ocean, sometimes storms, sometimes a very beautiful mirror-like peace, sukkha refers instead to the depths of the ocean, far beneath the waves on the surface, a depth of being that can remain stable throughout all these different changing states. It also includes a sense of wisdom in understanding the qualities of that state and distinguishing it from pleasure.

Pleasure is a sensation that, depending upon object, time, and circumstances, changes into a neutral state and sometimes into disgust. There is an element of tiredness in it. If you listen to the even most beautiful music for twenty-four hours, it becomes exhausting. It changes its nature. It's not something that the more you experience it, the deeper and more fulfilling it grows.

Sukkha, however, is the opposite. It is a way of being that is cultivated and grows deeper. It is associated with a cluster of qualities such as inner strength, inner freedom, compassion, and altruistic love. It's a way of being that is therefore less vulnerable to outer circumstances, although outer conditions influence it. But the more you experience it and understand what leads to the flourishing of that inner well-being, the clearer, deeper, and more stable it becomes. It is optimal in the sense that it becomes not second nature but your real nature.

Sukkha requires that one cease distorting reality. If one takes for permanent that which is ephemeral, if one believes that at the core of our being there is an autonomous self when there is none, if one confuses mere pleasurable sensations for lasting happiness, one is misconstruing reality, and that will cause suffering. Seen in this way, ignorance, delusion, and invalid cognition turn out to be the root cause of suffering.

We can immediately see how this relates to a sense of fear and insecurity. If you identify with and depend on the ups and downs, it's like waves breaking at the shore. Sometimes you are elated, surfing on top of the wave. Sometimes you crash on the rocks and are depressed. You need sukkha, that sense of inner well-being, precisely to not experience this feeling of insecurity.

Sukkha also relates to the notion of self-importance. An exacerbated self-importance that brings everything back to your own concerns is actually one of the main sources of insecurity. If you are always concerned about yourself, you are constantly a target of all the arrows. It's not just two arrows, it's a thousand arrows—of jealousy, resentment, hatred—all aimed at that feeling of self-importance. Hence the feeling of insecurity. That's why genuine confidence comes from somehow breaking that limited bubble of self-centeredness. When there is no more target, one can be genuinely self-confident. This has nothing to do with triumphant ego, but rather with being attuned to reality and understanding interdependence. The result is less insecurity.

In deep anguish or anxiety, there is also a failure to recognize or appreciate the potential for change that comes with an altruistic sense of connection with others and a deep compassion that makes you ready to act for the benefit of others. Identifying that potential within ourselves offers a great sense of direction and hope. It's an antidote to hopelessness. When you feel you're dropping into the bottomless pit of depression, you need that ledge that Helen's patient spoke about, from which you can progress further. The ledge is the identification of this potential for change. According to Buddhist tradition, we all have that potential. It is really the deepest nature of our mind. We give the example of the nugget of gold that is unchanged even in the mud, or the sun behind the clouds, which can always be rediscovered when the clouds blow away. In that sense, it is possible to actualize the flourishing of well-being. So sukkha connects the notion of well-being with the problem of excessive self-importance, and with the anxiety and anguish stemming from it, into a broader picture that is at the heart of the Buddhist path.

Bennett Shapiro: Coming back to Wolf's question about how the brain knows when it's arrived at "truth" or a "correct" view of things, I presume that you're speaking about an internal sense of the clouds suddenly clearing, a sense that you actually have arrived at that place.

Matthieu Ricard: Of course, it is not sudden. Hence the need to increase one's wisdom through analytic meditation and contemplative meditation over time.

Bennett Shapiro: Father Keating, you've been thinking about these intersections for a long time, and certainly these issues of how to deal with the self are part of your tradition as well.

Father Keating: It's been a wonderful learning experience for me to hear these experts in various health areas explain disease and the brain and other such things. I especially identify with their openness of mind and their openness to the spiritual dimension of the human condition. It has been mentioned, but I'd like to reinforce it by saying that for four hundred years, religion and science have been at one another's throat, if they got that close. I see your work, especially in this conference, as getting a toe, so to speak, in the door that has separated us. I engage in a great deal of interreligious dialogue, and I now see that science is also a religion of sorts and has its own dogmas and rituals. So I deeply welcome the invitation to participate in a deep dialogue with science.

In the Christian perspective, the early fathers of the Church accepted two books of revelation. One was the sacred scriptures, and the other was nature. Nature is a revelation of God, just as valid as the gifts of the prophets of the Old and New Testaments. The work of science and the discoveries of technology are revelations of God to us today. The expansion, depth, and breadth of research going on are telling me more about God than almost anything else, because I've already read the scriptures. What I'm interested in is finding out who God is. Einstein said that nature and science are God's thoughts. In their own way, scientists are just as much on the spiritual journey as we are in the monastery, as far as I can see.

To put this in the context of all the Abrahamic religions, the Garden of Eden, however mythological it is, communicates very profound truths about human nature. The great temptation in the Garden of Eden was that Adam and Eve were tempted to become God, or to be God's equal. This central drama of the human condition comes down to this: Do you want to become God on God's terms or on your own terms? If we become God on our own terms, then we're out of paradise. We're out of happiness, we're out of health, and we don't become God at all.

This reveals that the truth of human nature is really an ultimate desire to be happy. That translates into holistic health and sets up a context in which we can understand the ills of the human condition—body, soul, and spirit—that are part of our common experience. How this comes about is very significant for the health professions. If we're looking to become God on our own terms, we are very sick indeed. Our illusion is that if we obtain certain things, we'll be healthy or happy. It doesn't happen because this isn't how reality works.

As a result of being tossed out of the Garden of Eden, three things happened, at least symbolically, to the human race. It became sunk in illusion: it has no idea where true happiness is to be found. Hence, the second effect: we seek happiness in the wrong places, and this is the source of illness. Finally, if the human race is ever wise enough to find where true happiness might lie, it's too weak to do anything about it. One of the deep issues with trying to become God or happy or healthy is to be willing to accept that weakness and be content with being limited—to feel the need for the support of others and to feel accountable for all other members of the human race who are seeking happiness in the wrong places.

This is the gift of deep, transconceptual meditation. This is why it is so important. It opens us to reality before we start thinking. Not that thinking isn't a great advance over the situation of our mammalian ancestors, but deep meditation is a gift that allows us to go beyond thinking to the intuitive presence of reality, to the bonding that takes place beyond rational consciousness and can best be described as love. Love is the capacity to know at the deepest level of knowledge, beyond knowledge of a conceptual kind.

In this context, the Christian ascetic and mystical tradition talks of seeking God on God's own terms. You can call God by other names, and He still is God, or She is still God, or It is still God. And God suffers from worse names than God. The contemplative vision shows God as close to us—closer than we are to ourselves—and within that vision our whole

197

being emerges from this ground or presence. The great contribution of the Christian religion, it seems to me, is that this presence is tender, loving, motherly, concerned, caring, health-giving—all the aspects of love we know rolled into one and given totally gratuitously. And God as our host invites us to treat the rest of humanity as if we were their host. In other words, we are to pass on the great goodness that we are constantly receiving.

I might just mention that Contemplative Outreach is an organization that is designed to recover the Christian contemplative tradition from earlier times. This tradition has fallen somewhat into neglect, desuetude, and positive opposition in some places, so most Christians need to be converted. I certainly include myself because, in the order I belong to, we take a vow of continuing conversion. That is a way of saying that we don't take ourselves as a fixed reality, that we think of the self as *not* a fixed point of reference. Hence, it can change, it can grow, and its capacity for truth and love and happiness is constantly expanding. I think Buddhists would call this compassion.

In my opportunities to dialogue with the other great spiritual traditions, I see something emerging that is beyond interreligious dialogue. It might be called interspiritual dialogue. This is the common bond experienced by those who are committed to the transformative process. Contemplative Outreach tries to make the monastic vision available to people living in the world or working in intense active ministries, and a resource of strength for those engaged in very difficult ministries.

The heart of the discipline of Christian meditation is silence, which is not emptiness, but listening at a deeper level than the ears or even the heart can reach. It's listening to that energy out of which everything emerges, which is both energy and no energy, which is nothing and everything at the same time, and which invites us into its own immense freedom—if we will just sit down and shut up for maybe twenty minutes. It doesn't matter how we sit. What does matter is that doing so discontinues habits of looking for happiness in the wrong place. It is thinking that sustains that—and makes us all quite ill.

Alan Wallace: I'd like to bring together two themes. One is from the very eminent historian Daniel Boorstin, who wrote a history of humanity's discoveries over the last five thousand years: *The Discoverers*.[98] In the preface to that book, he commented that the greatest impediment to discovery throughout the whole of human history was not ignorance, but the illusion of knowledge—the belief that we already know something that, in fact, is merely an assumption. As long as we're holding on to the illusion of knowledge, it impedes breaking through and gaining actual knowledge.

A second theme is from His Holiness, when he said that it may be impossible to determine whether any isolated moment of cognition, an awareness of any sort, is valid within itself. You can determine whether it is valid in interrelationship with other moments of cognition. Or you can evaluate whether your own cognitions are valid with respect to another person, say Thupten Jinpa: "Am I seeing that glass correctly?" Well, I'll ask him.

If we take that as a metaphor, we have a moment of cognition called "neurobiology for the last thirty years," which has its own perspective. In that perspective there is certainly a lot of knowledge. There may also be illusions of knowledge, for example, about the nature of consciousness. Is consciousness purely a function of the brain? Good question. If one is focusing entirely on the brain, then what other conclusion could one possibly draw? On the other hand, if you spent those thirty years, or three thousand years, primarily studying mental phenomena, you might draw a different conclusion.

The simple point here is that multiple theories, or multiple moments of awareness, may best be validated when they are brought into conjunction with moments of awareness or perspectives that are radically different. Whether our perspective is Christianity, Buddhism, the philosophy of Greek antiquity, or modern neurobiology, the way forward may be to overcome the illusions of knowledge by engaging deeply, respectfully, and humbly with people who share radically different visions.

I think there's a common assumption from a secular perspective that the religions of the world cancel themselves out in terms of any truth claims: Christianity, Buddhism, Hinduism, and Taoism say many different things on many fronts, so when you shuffle them all together, they all collapse into nothing. In that view, the only moment of cognition that seems to be left standing is science, with nothing to bounce off of because religions have canceled each other out.

It's also often believed that the contemplative traditions feel they already know the answers. You set out on your contemplative path and are guided to the right answer. If you deviate from that, your teacher brings you back and says, "Not that way. We already know the right answer. Keep on meditating until you get to the right answer." That is completely incompatible with the spirit of scientific inquiry, which seeks information currently thought to be unknown, and is therefore open to something fresh.

As I put these various problems together in my mind, a solution seems to rise up, which is a strong return to empiricism and clarity. What don't we know and what do we know? It's very hard to find that out when we only engage with people who have similar mentalities to our own. As Father Thomas suggested, Christianity needs to return to a spirit of empiricism, to the contemplative experience, rather than resting with all the "right" answers from doctrine. The same goes for Buddhism. In this regard I'm deeply inspired by the words of William James: "Let empiricism once become associated with religion, as hitherto, through some strange misunderstanding, it has been associated with irreligion, and I believe that a new era of religion as well as philosophy will be ready to begin . . . I fully believe that such an empiricism is a more natural ally than dialectics ever were, or can be, of the religious life."[99] We may then find there are indeed profound convergences among multiple contemplative traditions operating out of very different initial frameworks: the Bible, the sutras, the Vedas, and so forth. When we go to the deepest experiential level, there may be universal contemplative truths that the Christians, the Buddhists, and the Taoists have each found in their laboratories. If there is some convergence, these may be some of the most important truths that human beings can ever access.

Bennett Shapiro: Alan, that was so beautifully said, and it stresses the kind of empiricism that we're trying to achieve in these dialogues. We're trying to be open-minded, to realize that we don't know as much as we think we know, and to be wary. I completely agree that the biggest danger, in medicine as well, is thinking that you know more than you actually know. When you make assumptions that go far beyond your knowledge base, that's when you really start doing harm. For everything that we're engaged in as a collective group, this concept is central.

The issue of the essential goodness of humans and the quality of compassion has come up repeatedly in these discussions. We seem to understand these as an important foundation in helping us achieve closer connections with others. In recent years, Sharon Salzberg has spent a lot of her time engaging in compassion-related meditations and teaching compassion to large groups of laypeople who are not necessarily Buddhists. Sharon, I wonder whether, in this mix of ideas, you might cast a few thoughts in that direction.

Sharon Salzberg: When I was looking through the notes I've taken throughout this conference, two words appeared on every page: "compassion" and "helplessness." Every speaker either used the word "helplessness" or said something that made me think of it. The recognition of how much we need to care as a natural outcome of seeing the world in a certain way comes together very powerfully with the recognition of how little control we have over making things be the way we want. Even though compassion is held up as an ideal in the West, it's also often discounted, especially in its manifestation as kindness. It's almost a secondary virtue—if we can't be brilliant, or brave or wonderful at least we can try to be kind—as though it is in some way meager or mediocre. But in the reality of people's day-to-day lives, I think kindness is a tremendous thread that's of great importance not only for living in a better way, but for having a bigger view of what life is.

I'm going to be teaching a five-week class on compassion here in Washington, DC, next year. At first I thought I'd make it a requirement of the class that you have to engage in some kind of service. You have to volunteer at a soup kitchen or a homeless shelter or do something like that. Then the organizer of the class asked me, "What if somebody is taking care of an ill parent? Does that count, or is that not enough? Do they have to go out and do something special?" I was embarrassed, because I thought of how many people I know who are taking care of an ill parent or a troubled child or a sick friend. That really is the challenge. It is something we confront in our lives every day. What is compassion? What is kindness? How can I live them?

Coming back to the issue of helplessness, the teachings talk about different levels of compassion and different kinds of compassion. There is the compassion where we feel we can do something about the situation, and the compassion where we feel we can't do anything. I wonder if His Holiness would speak about that, because it is such a powerful consideration. Does compassion change to something else in those circumstances, or is it supported by our wisdom, our insight into emptiness? What sustains compassion when we feel helpless?

HH Dalai Lama: As you are aware, in the Buddhist texts there is a recognition of a type of compassion that is reinforced and complemented by the faculty of wisdom. In the texts this is sometimes referred to as "compassion endowed with the wisdom of emptiness." The idea is that when compassion is complemented and reinforced by the faculty of wisdom, the individual has the ability not only to empathize, but also to understand the causes and conditions that led to that suffering, and to envision the possibility of freedom from that state. Therefore, this compassion complemented by wisdom is thought to be very powerful and much more effective. It is a more forceful state of mind.

Generally, compassion is characterized as a state of mind that wishes to see the other free of suffering. In that sense, an individual who experiences compassion can also feel a sense of helplessness. That type of compassion may be primarily a form of empathy, with the wish that other persons be free of suffering, but it can be more powerful when it's not simply a wish to see others free from suffering, but also has the added dimension of willingness to help others be free of suffering. Here, it is wisdom or intelligence that plays the pivotal role in allowing a compassionate wish to translate into altruistic action, and it is a more powerful type of compassion.

The texts also speak of boundless compassion and great compassion. Great compassion is defined as the forceful compassion that gives rise to the altruistic aspiration to seek enlightenment for the benefit of all. According to the Mahayana Buddhist texts, when an individual has generated great compassion within himself or herself, then Buddha nature has been awakened or activated.

Richard Davidson: Your Holiness, this has been a very wonderful meeting, and I'd like to express our gratitude to you for spending so much time with us. I mentioned a theme at the very outset, which has been preserved through much of the meeting, and I'd like to come back to that now. There is a remarkable convergence between a key insight that has emerged both in modern neuroscience and from the contemplative traditions, which is that virtuous qualities of the human mind can be regarded as skills that can be cultivated. The fact of brain plasticity provides a foundation for understanding how the cultivation of these qualities may be supported by the brain and how the brain may change in response to these practices.

I find an increased receptivity to these ideas when I talk about this work, which I have freely done since I met Your Holiness more than ten years ago; you've been an inspiration to do that. The scientific research is beginning to play a role in the increasing acceptance of the idea that we're not stuck where we are. We're not stuck at our set points; rather, the mind can be transformed. I envision a time when schoolchildren in the United States and other Western cultures will be required to attend not only PE, which stands for physical education, but also a class called ME, for mental education. Wouldn't that be wonderful?

Your participation and your involvement is so inspiring in helping us spread this important message. I think the scientific work we're doing provides one small piece of that larger message.

I'd also like to take this opportunity to acknowledge that Jon and I go back thirty years. We first met in Cambridge, where I was a graduate student and Jon was in the middle of a career transition from being a molecular biologist to becoming a meditation teacher. He helped provide me with the beginning of my alternative education in mental training, starting in the 1970s. So for us to be working together in this way now is a wonderful coming full circle. I don't think either of us envisioned that we would be in this situation today, but it feels so perfect that we are.

I would also like to take this opportunity to express my gratitude to Adam Engle, who has worked tirelessly on behalf of all of us for so many years, We would not have these meetings without his dedication and fine work. It is wonderful that you are here, that you exist on this planet to make this possible, and we're all so grateful.

Jon Kabat-Zinn: Your Holiness, my heart is full at this moment. I feel a tremendous sense of gratitude and happiness for the opportunities that you continually afford us to look more deeply into the nature of reality, to remind ourselves how little we understand of reality or of ourselves. Rather than being frightened by that condition, we can realize that it is an incredible invitation to part the veil of our own highly conditioned and habitual seeing, an invitation to see beyond those limitations to a much deeper actuality of who and how we are, individually and collectively.

It is enormously moving to me that you work ceaselessly around the world to bring the energy of compassion and wisdom to humanity, making house call after house call, from the house here at the Constitution Hall to the White House, and on to the next, continually embodying in your being what it might mean for each of us to be truly human. I know that people put you on a pedestal, and I know that you have said many times that you are simply a Buddhist monk, but none of us here has a snowball's chance in hell of becoming the Dalai Lama! However, we do potentially have a chance—that very fleeting chance called a human lifetime—to move closer to who we already are. So much of the time we live in our thoughts and delusions about how things are and who we are, rather than inhabiting what Francisco Varela called "embodied mindful awareness."

In closing, I'd like to respond to Father Thomas's very inclusive invitation to remember what it means to love, to be in love, and to be love. A few lines from Wordsworth's "Prelude" come to mind: "There is a dark inscrutable workmanship that reconciles discordant elements, makes them move in one society."[100] I think of the continual flux, the deconstructing and cohering of patterns of connection in the brain, moment by moment. Whether you call it Tao or dharma or God or I-don't-have-the-slightest-idea, there is certainly a sense that we are participating in something quite extraordinary and mysterious.

This time together has been like a bell ringing for five sessions over two and half days. The bell has now rung, but the reverberations have the potential to go out infinitely. We do not know what the consequences are of having eavesdropped on this conversation in His Holiness's portable living room, but whatever the consequences may be, they will have something to do with all the questions that didn't get answered.

The challenge is to ask where those questions come from in the first place, and what your job on the planet is, whether it has to do with children, with trauma, with the military, with government, or with something else. The challenge is to ask, "What is my job on this planet, in this moment, given who I am and everything I know—including whatever has come from this dialogue? Might this inquiry begin to cohere and synchronize for us, individually and collectively, into some deeper manifestation of what it might actually mean to belong to *Homo sapiens sapiens*, the species that knows, and knows that it knows, in other words, the species of awareness and awareness of awareness?" Or will we go back to sleep on our way home?

I was so touched by what Richie said, and I want to bow to him for holding seemingly different worlds in a way that truly has heart. I value our friendship tremendously and am deeply appreciative of the opportunity to have been able to work together to develop this meeting and host it together.

Adam Engle: You guys have stolen a little bit of my thunder. I was going to talk about your relationship over the last thirty-five years.

Jon Kabat-Zinn: You can do the third-person approach. We've just done the first-person approach.

Adam Engle: Your Holiness, I'd like to reflect together on the improbability of us being here today. It continually amazes me.

His Holiness was born in one of the most remote regions on the planet and has become one of the preeminent spiritual leaders on the planet—and is also dedicated steadfastly to this interchange between science and spirituality. I find that so incredible, and I want to thank you on behalf of everyone here, and everyone who has ever been involved in the Mind and Life Institute, for drawing us together in this joint quest for the benefit of humanity.

I'd also like to thank someone who isn't publicly thanked a lot: your brother, Tendzin Choegyal. He was the first person I spoke to in His Holiness's entourage about the possibility of what has become the Mind and Life Dialogues. He has been a steadfast friend and supporter of the Mind and Life Institute from that day on, as well as a very close personal friend. Thanks also to the members of the Private Office, who put up with my constant badgering to try to get on His Holiness's schedule.

Richie and Jon have already acknowledged their past history together for thirty-five years. It's another improbability that two guys who met when they were graduate students have stayed together all this time, have led this endeavor over the last decade, and will continue to do so. It's a pleasure to work with you both.

I'd also like to acknowledge and thank all of the presenters and panelists. You have no idea how much effort they have put into making this happen. It takes countless meetings, conference calls, and phone calls, and many days of preparation.

Finally, I would like to close with a Buddhist practice of dedicating merit. Whatever benefit and merit may have arisen here, we dedicate it for the benefit of all beings.

EPILOGUE

ADVANCES IN BASIC AND CLINICAL RESEARCH ON MEDITATION IN THE FIVE YEARS FOLLOWING MIND AND LIFE XIII: 2006–2011

The meeting upon which this book is based was held in November 2005. Since that time, and in part as a result of our meeting, research on meditation has flourished and is continuing its exponential rise. In this concluding section, we highlight what we consider to be some of the most important findings in basic and clinical research, the methodological challenges associated with this phase of the rigorous study of meditative practices, and questions that this new wave of research has ushered in. We have deliberately chosen not to be exhaustive. There are a number of reviews since 2005 that focus on various components of this literature.[101] Our purpose here is to highlight the most promising new findings in this emerging field and then discuss some of the challenges now facing it.

BASIC RESEARCH

This section outlines basic research findings that are aimed at deepening our understanding of the phenomena associated with meditative practices, and their underlying biological mechanisms.

Cognitive and Attentional Function

In the past five years, considerable progress has been made in characterizing how various forms of meditation change basic cognitive and affective processes and their underlying neural circuits. For example, one study examined the impact of three months of intensive vipassana practice in a retreat setting and reported on behavioral and neural changes associated with the attentional blink, in which heightened response to an initial stimulus prevents subjects from seeing a second stimulus.[102] This effect may be due to a kind of excitement about or overinvestment in detecting the initial target that clouds the ability to see the subsequent target. Prior to the retreat, there were no differences between the meditators and age- and gender-matched control participants. However, after three months of practice, the meditators had less attentional blink, detecting the second target stimulus with significantly greater accuracy. These behavioral changes were accompanied by measurable changes in brain function. The three months of intensive practice apparently increased the meditators' ability to allocate attention in a more balanced way, improving their performance on the task.

Another study looked at response time variability on a selective attention task with the same participants.[103] Again, the three months of intensive practice improved performance, significantly reducing variability in response times. Response time variability is a particularly interesting aspect of accomplishing tasks that require selective attention, since greater variability is closely associated with attention deficit/hyperactivity disorder. The reduction in response time variability was associated with a striking change in brain function. In a brain that is maximally receptive and attentive to stimuli, the phase of ongoing neural oscillations synchronizes with the onset of the stimulus. It is as if the brain is ready and attentive, so that the occurrence of an external stimulus to which the person attends is immediately apprehended by this phase-locking process. In this study, researchers reported that the reduction in response time variability was associated with an enhancement of phase-locking between cortical rhythms and the external stimulus to which participants were instructed to attend.

The Shamatha Project, mentioned by Alan Wallace during his presentation, examined the impact of three months of intensive training in a concentration meditation practice known as shamatha, comparing performance on a sustained attention task between the meditators and a wait-list control group.[104] The training resulted in significant improvements in perceptual sensitivity and vigilance.

Improvements in visuospatial processing and working memory have also been reported for a meditation training that was much less intensive than the Shamatha Project, and in which participants were initially new to meditation. In one study, participants were randomly assigned to four sessions of either meditation training or listening to a recorded book.[105] The meditation training was based upon the work of Alan Wallace, who was the meditation teacher in the Shamatha Project.[106] Researchers reported that this meditation training led to significantly greater enhancements in visuospatial processing and working memory than the control group experienced.

An unusual study of selective improvements in cognitive function compared performance between similarly advanced practitioners of two different styles of Tibetan Buddhist meditation: deity yoga, which involves visualizing a complex and multicolored three-dimensional image of a Tibetan deity, and open presence meditation, which involves cultivating evenly distributed attention that is not directed to any particular object or experience.[107] The effect of these very different forms of meditation on visuospatial processing was measured before and after a twenty-minute period of meditation practice. The deity yoga practice led to substantial improvements on both a mental rotation task and a visual memory task compared with the open presence meditation. These results indicate that a short period of practice is sufficient to induce changes that persist into a subsequent task period and selectively enhances tasks that depend upon visual information processing.

Alterations in Brain Function and Structure

An important recent study on the impact of meditation on the neural processing of pain found reduced activation in executive, evaluative, and emotion-related brain regions during exposure to thermal pain among a group of Zen practitioners compared with nonmeditating controls.[108] Moreover, the most experienced meditators exhibited the largest reductions in activation in these regions. Interestingly, the meditators simultaneously showed enhanced activation in primary pain processing regions, including the anterior cingulate, thalamus, and insula. Reductions in functional connectivity between executive and pain-related regions of the brain predicted lower pain sensitivity among the meditators. These findings imply a functional uncoupling of the cognitive-evaluative and sensory-discriminative dimensions of pain among the Zen practitioners, a phenomenon originally observed and described in patients with chronic pain conditions trained in MBSR.[109]

A study of an eight-week MBSR intervention using functional magnetic resonance imaging demonstrated changes in the activity of two distinct neural pathways in the brain associated with self-referencing.[110] The narrative focus pathway is associated with linking of experiences across time. It appears to be anatomically coextensive with the medial prefrontal cortex and the so-called default network,[111] which has been shown to be associated with narrative-generating mind-wandering and perhaps plays a role in the generation of narrative.[112] The second neural pathway that demonstrated changes was the experiential focus pathway, which seems to be related to self-referencing of direct somatic experience in the present moment. While the narrative focus pathway is associated with activity in the medial prefrontal cortex, the experiential focus pathway is associated with a right-lateralized network that includes the lateral prefrontal cortex and viscerosomatic regions such as the insula, the secondary somatosensory cortex, and the inferior parietal lobe.

The eight-week MBSR training resulted in marked and pervasive reductions in activity in the circuit associated with narrative focus and increased activation in the network associated with experiential focus. This suggests that these two very different forms of self-referencing, which often occur at the same time, can be uncoupled through mindfulness training, a finding that may be of clinical importance in loosening the hold of self-centered narratives associated with depressive rumination and other unconscious habits of self-preoccupation and absorption that cause and amplify suffering.

It is possible that future studies will show that mindfulness training can be instrumental in shifting the default mode from distracted mind-wandering (what some term the "doing" mode of mind) to one of mindful awareness (the "being mode" of mind).[113] Moreover, with deepening practice, mindfulness training might play a role in fostering a shift from a transitory state to a more enduring and robust trait, a way of being grounded in present-moment embodied experience rather than being caught in an elaborate cognitive self-narrative characteristic of depressive rumination, chronic anxiety, daydreaming, and self-absorbed fantasizing.

Building on this finding, a subsequent study examined the impact of MBSR training on the processing of negative affect.[114] The study used a paradigm that induced negative affect by provoking sadness. Once again, this affective shift was found to recruit widespread networks known to be involved in self-referential processing. The group trained in MBSR showed a diminished neural response in the narrative focus network and augmented activity in the experiential focus network compared to the wait-list control group. Despite equivalent levels of self-reported sadness, the MBSR participants showed greater activation of the lateral neural circuits associated with experiential focus—those associated with visceral and somatosensory processes and the perception of bodily sensations. The recruitment of these neural regions was associated with decreased depression scores among the MBSR participants.

These findings suggest pathways through which mindfulness training may beneficially influence the processing of negative emotion and alter the neural circuitry through which sadness itself is experienced. Novices who experienced temporary sad moods activated the narrative focus network: brain areas that treated their sadness as a problem to be analyzed and solved. People trained in MBSR, on the other hand, activated the experiential focus network: brain areas that provided feedback about what sadness felt like in the body. At the level of conscious experience, practicing mindfulness seems to allow individuals to see that it is possible to take a wholly different approach to the endless cycles of mental strategizing and affliction that are part and parcel of depression and anxiety.

In a recent study that used magnetoencephalography (MEG) to examine changes in the alpha rhythm during the anticipation of a subtle sensory

cue, researchers found that in response to a cue that instructed participants to attend to a hand versus a foot, eight weeks of MBSR training led
to significantly enhanced localized cortical responses during the anticipation period compared with controls who were not trained in MBSR.[115]
This finding suggests that specific changes in the brain occur in relation
to specific attention to the body with meditation training.

A major new area of interest that has emerged in recent years involves
the question of whether systematic training in meditation may be associated with actual structural changes in the brain. Basic research on
neuroplasticity certainly suggests the possibility of structural changes in
response to mental training. However, it is only in the past several years
that a sufficient body of evidence has accumulated to strongly suggest that
such changes do in fact occur. In a recent randomized trial,[116] Sara Lazar
and her colleagues demonstrated increases in gray matter density in several brain regions critical for learning, memory, and emotion regulation,
including the hippocampus and posterior cingulate, following MBSR
training. Another related study from Lazar's group linked reductions in
self-reported perceived stress produced by MBSR to decreases in gray matter density in the right basolateral amygdala.[117] This is the first report of
structural changes in the amygdala following MBSR training. Future
research may determine the extent to which other affective changes
reported with MBSR might be associated with changes in the size of the
amygdala.

Alterations in Autonomic, Immune, and Endocrine Function

The effects of meditation on the autonomic nervous system are likely
to be complex and to vary with the type of meditation practice. In 2006,
two studies[118] investigated the impact of body scan–based meditation practices derived from MBSR on a range of autonomic functions. The first
study compared a group using the body scan meditation as taught in
MBSR to a group using progressive muscle relaxation and a wait-list control. The second study compared effects of the body scan meditation
practice to a control condition in which the same participants listened to
a popular novel on audiotape. In both studies, during the body scan

meditation, participants showed significantly higher respiratory sinus arrhythmia, an index that reflects effects on cardiac control by the parasympathetic nervous system (sometimes known as "rest and digest," in contrast to the fight-or-flight functions of the sympathetic nervous system). In the second study only, a marker sensitive to sympathetic nervous system influence on the heart was measured. Interestingly, this study found a significant increase in sympathetic nervous system influence on the heart with meditation compared with the control condition. Collectively, the findings from this report suggest increases in both parasympathetic and sympathetic cardiac activity during the body scan meditation practice among novice practitioners. This is a particularly interesting and important finding since the parasympathetic nervous system and sympathetic nervous system are usually inversely related but mindfulness meditation appeared to activate both branches of the autonomic nervous system simultaneously.

A recent report from the Shamatha Project[119] measured telomerase activity following a three-month retreat emphasizing shamatha practice compared with a wait-list control group. Telomeres are repeated DNA sequences at the end of the chromosomes that protect critical genetic information within the chromosome from being damaged, and telomerase is the enzyme that extends and/or restores these sequences at the ends of chromosomes. Telomerase activity is of major interest because lower levels, along with reductions in telomere length, have been linked to accelerated rates of biological aging in the face of unremitting stress.[120] At the end of the retreat, telomerase activity was significantly greater among the shamatha practitioners compared to the controls. The researchers also reported observing complex relationships between changes on a number of self-reported personality dimensions (such as neuroticism) and telomerase activity between groups. Those retreat practitioners who showed the greatest increases in perceived control and greater decreases in neuroticism after the retreat showed the largest increases in telomerase activity.

Mindfulness and related practices that emphasize attention to bodily sensations might be expected to enhance visceral awareness. Objective methods for measuring visceral self-perception, or interoceptive awareness as it is sometimes called, have been developed. Moreover, in neuroscientific studies, individual differences in visceral self-perception have been found to be associated with activation in the insula.[121] The most commonly used task reflects the extent to which participants can accurately perceive their own heartbeat. One study that used this task[122] compared seventeen practitioners of kundalini meditation, a practice involving breath manipulation that places emphasis on somatic awareness; thirteen practitioners of a Tibetan meditation that emphasizes open monitoring, in which practitioners nonreactively focus on the moment-to-moment content of their experience[123]; and seventeen nonmeditating controls. Meditators in each tradition had a minimum of fifteen years of daily practice. This study found no evidence of superior heartbeat detection in either group of meditators compared with controls. Participants in this study were also asked to rate how well they believed they performed. The meditators consistently rated their performance higher than nonmeditators did, despite absolutely no difference in objective performance. The findings from this study are instructive in underscoring the limitations of meditation in producing certain types of effects, such as unusual sensitivity to bodily states. They also highlight potential differences in self-view and worldview that may have led the meditators to believe they were superior in spite of objective evidence to the contrary.

CLINICAL RESEARCH

Among the significant developments since the 2005 meeting has been the continued investigation and spread of mindfulness-based cognitive therapy, an intervention modeled on MBSR that Zindel Segal described in his presentation in session 3. This intervention is now recommended by the National Health Service in the United Kingdom for people with a history of three or more episodes of major depressive disorder.[124] MBCT, which was designed to help recovered but recurrently depressed patients develop mindfulness strategies for relating differently to patterns of thinking that induce depression, significantly decreases the risk of relapse and recurrence.[125] MBCT emphasizes daily practice of formal and informal mindfulness meditation practices, including mindful yoga. These practices may also serve as ideal constituents of an ongoing maintenance strategy, particularly in regard to depressive rumination.

In an important new study,[126] Zindel Segal and his colleagues tested eighty-four patients with a diagnosis of major depressive disorder who were currently in remission following treatment with an antidepressant medication. These patients were randomly assigned to one of three conditions: discontinuing the antidepressants and attending eight weekly group sessions of MBCT; continuing with their therapeutic dose of antidepressant; or discontinuing active medication and being transitioned onto placebo. The main outcome measure was relapse into a depressive episode. The findings revealed that MBCT and continued medication were equivalent in protecting against relapse compared with placebo. Thus, the study importantly showed that MBCT can be considered a medically equivalent alternative to medication for patients at risk for major depressive relapse who do not wish to continue on antidepressants.

Another study recently examined the impact of MBSR on emotion regulation in patients with social anxiety disorder.[127] It found that MBSR led to improvements in symptoms of anxiety and depression, and in self-esteem in a small group of these patients. Following the MBSR intervention, participants were monitored during a task probing negative self-beliefs while they were also engaging in either a breath-focused attention task or a distraction task. Functional magnetic resonance imaging showed decreased negative emotional experience and decreased activation in the amygdala during the breath-focused task.

Variants of MBSR have been developed to specifically address substance abuse and craving. Mindfulness-based relapse prevention (MBRP) is the most well-developed intervention of this sort.[128] In the most comprehensive study of MBRP for patients with substance use disorder,[129] 168 patients were randomly assigned to either MBRP or treatment as usual, which consisted of counseling and educational information. Among patients receiving treatment as usual, the experience of craving was associated with both depressive symptoms and substance use. However, MBRP significantly changed the relationship between craving and depression so that when feelings of craving arose, they no longer automatically triggered depression, and these changes predicted reduced substance use four months after the intervention. These findings indicate that while MBRP does not directly affect substance use, it does decrease the link between craving and depression, and this in turn may affect subsequent substance use. Clearly, additional research is required to tease apart these complex effects and to determine whether preexisting individual differences are associated with differential response to interventions such as MBRP.

A recent study indicated that brief mindfulness training for cigarette smokers resulted in greater reductions in cigarette use following a four-week mindfulness-based treatment and at a seventeen-week follow-up compared to individuals randomized to an American Lung Association Freedom from Smoking treatment. Mindfulness was shown to directly reduce craving itself in this study.[130]

METHODOLOGICAL CHALLENGES

As several recent comprehensive reviews of selective segments of the scientific literature on the impact of meditation reveal, the methodological shortcomings of the extant research are considerable. For example, a major 2007 report on the health effects of meditation commissioned by the National Center for Complementary and Alternative Medicine reached the following conclusion: "Scientific research on meditation practices does not appear to have a common theoretical perspective and is characterized by poor methodological quality. Firm conclusions on the effects of meditation practices in healthcare cannot be drawn based on the available evidence. Future research on meditation practices must be more rigorous in the design and execution of studies and in the analysis and reporting of results."[131] We wholeheartedly agree with this assessment of the field at this point in time.

There are numerous critical methodological issues germane to the scientific study of clinical interventions, particularly psychological interventions, but here we focus on a few that are unique to research on meditation. One of the most critical is the choice of control groups for intervention studies. For example, what would be a proper control group for MBSR? This question is becoming increasingly relevant. It is clear that a wait-list control design, while a perfectly appropriate choice for earlier studies, is now no longer sufficient, since there are many features of MBSR interventions that are not specific to the meditation practices themselves but might contribute to changes in standard outcome measures. Comparison conditions that match the MBSR condition for variables such as group process, enthusiasm of the instructor, belief that the intervention will produce beneficial change, length of home practice, and so on are necessary to conclusively establish that the meditation practices per se are responsible for the measured outcomes. As of this writing, no published study has adopted such rigorous comparison conditions. However, Richard Davidson's laboratory has developed such a comparison condition and will soon publish the results of several studies that make use of this comparison group.[132] For the present purposes, we can summarize by saying that there were no significant differences observed on any of the standard self-report outcome measures between MBSR participants and a rigorous comparison group that controlled for the range of nonspecific factors listed above. However, and interestingly, there were numerous differences between the groups on biological measures and on responsivity to pain, with all biological measures showing positive effects in the MBSR condition.

Other critical methodological issues concern measurement of practice time and assessment of past meditation experience. For the latter, the field critically needs a formal structured interview for use with different meditation traditions that would yield reliable measures of past practice. Measuring practice time within a study is somewhat more complicated since there are many opportunities for informal practice that might not get incorporated into people's reports of their practice time. Also, it has not been established that individuals report practice time reliably. While we are not suggesting that people would consciously dissimulate about their practice time, it is well-known that many individuals show a propensity to present themselves in a positive light, and many of the meditation studies inevitably create an expectation that good subjects are those who practice as much as they are told to practice. We thus will ultimately need more objective measures of practice time. Richard Davidson's laboratory has been experimenting with the development of a "wired zafu," a meditation cushion equipped with a pressure-sensitive gauge to measure the amount of time a person is actually sitting on the cushion. Of course, such a measure is also fraught with problems since both formal and informal meditation practice can occur anywhere and need not take place on the cushion. Nor is time sitting on the cushion necessarily directly correlated with practice, much less with quality of practice or insight. Nevertheless, some attention to this issue is required in future research.

Of particular importance for studies of meditation practices that emphasize mindfulness is a behavioral measure of mindfulness. Self-report measures have uncertain validity. Moreover, individuals' ability to report on their internal experience may not be well developed, particularly in the early stages of meditation practice. Thus, self-report questionnaires may reflect a person's internal biases about the kinds of experiences "a mindful person" is supposed to have, rather than being a veridical report of actual interior experience. This is an area of vigorous debate and investigation at present.[133] A well-validated behavioral measure that takes these important issues into account would enable investigators to more systematically examine individual differences by determining if participants who show greater increases in the behavioral measure of mindfulness also show more improvements in the other outcome measures being assessed. This would place the field on a considerably firmer footing than it now occupies, since virtually all analytic efforts to characterize individual differences in mindfulness to date have relied on such self-report measures.

PROSPECTS FOR THE FUTURE

In this final section we point toward some promising trends on the horizon in both basic and clinical research on meditation. On the clinical side, we are beginning to better understand relations between the central circuitry of emotion and peripheral biology that may be relevant to health and to specific illnesses.[134] This growing knowledge provides a foundation for examining and understanding how different forms of meditation may influence the central circuitry of emotion and, in turn, have downstream consequences that are relevant to specific health outcomes. If a physical disorder can be influenced to one degree or another by psychosocial factors, we would expect that the brain would be involved in modulating the peripheral organ systems implicated in the disease, allowing for the possible influence on disease-relevant biology via modulation of central neural circuits through meditation. We expect that future studies of such physical diseases will be accompanied by measurements of brain function in addition to peripheral biological markers so that the changes in the brain that are most strongly related to changes in relevant symptoms and physiological processes can be ascertained. In this way, research on meditation can contribute to an overall better understanding of mind-brain-body interactions in both health and disease.

At the level of whole populations, research is critically needed to evaluate the impact of meditation on health care utilization. While there are anecdotal descriptions of decreased health care utilization among meditation practitioners, no rigorous studies have examined this issue. This kind of effort should ideally be guided by a health care economist and be conducted at multiple sites. If meditation is found to reduce health care utilization even by a few percentage points, it would have enormous economic consequences for health care, nationally and globally. This kind of information would provide a powerful incentive for government and insurance agencies to take meditative practices more seriously at the public health level. We hope that a well-designed and rigorous study of the effects of a meditation-based intervention on health care utilization will be undertaken as soon as possible.

While there have been a number of recent reports on the application of meditation in children, the literature is spotty, the interventions extremely varied, and the outcomes poorly measured.[135] However, the potential for intervention early in life to have a beneficial impact on specific conditions is high, given that neuroplasticity is likely to be greater, particularly during the preadolescent period. A recent preliminary study suggests that mindfulness meditation may have some promise in helping children with attention deficit/hyperactivity disorder.[136] The stakes could not be higher. Among teens between the ages of twelve and nineteen years, more than 75 percent of deaths are due to accidents (mostly motor vehicle accidents), homicide, or suicide.[137] Most of the motor vehicle accidents are caused by drugs or alcohol. Thus, methods of mental training that might help cultivate greater equanimity, emotional balance, and discernment prior to entering the adolescent risk period are critical, and might be potentially lifesaving. An appreciation of impermanence and not taking personally what is not personal are certainly critical elements of mindfulness training that might greatly benefit children and adolescents.

In terms of basic research, two major methodological and conceptual advances are likely to have dramatic impacts on the kinds of questions that can be asked about the impact of meditation practice in the future. One is epigenetics, the study of the factors that regulate gene expression. It has now been definitively established that environmental factors can regulate gene expression.[138] This raises the possibility that mental training can also regulate gene expression, though as yet no rigorous published studies have addressed this issue. There is preliminary evidence that relaxation procedures produce alterations in gene expression, though systematic comparisons with rigorous control groups have not yet been reported.[139] We expect that in the next few years a number of research groups will examine epigenetic changes produced by meditation. Though the cell types available for epigenetic study in the intact human are quite limited, the fact that meditation produces demonstrable changes in peripheral biology should provide some clues as to appropriate targets of epigenetic change. The glucocorticoid receptor gene is one obvious place to look, based on the groundbreaking studies in rats by Michael Meaney and his colleagues.[140]

The other major methodological and conceptual advance concerns the human connectome—the project to map the functional and structural connections of the human brain.[141] Methods are now available to characterize structural and functional connections between each volume element (that is, the three-dimension pixel known as a voxel) and every other voxel in the human brain. Such rich information might contain sufficient sensitivity to better characterize the impact of different forms of meditation on neural circuits. Rather than focusing analyses on isolated zones of activation, connectivity measures might provide much richer and more robust measures of circuit structure and function, which are likely to be of great relevance to understanding how meditation affects the mind and brain.

When the Mind and Life XIII meeting was held in 2005, the modern era of research on meditation was just beginning. The past five years have seen tremendously rapid progress in both basic and clinical research. We anticipate that the next five years will witness an even greater flowering of meditation-based clinical interventions and basic research, conducted at increasingly high levels of rigor in terms of hypothesis development, model building, research design (including choice of active control groups), brain and peripheral biological measures, and behavioral measures, as well as more precise descriptions of the meditation practices themselves. We anticipate that the coming years will be even more productive than those that are now behind us, and that meditation will move even further into the mainstream of neuroscience, psychology, and medicine, reflecting the spirit of the Mind and Life meeting of 2005 and the ever-deepening confluence of the streams of science and the meditative traditions.

Our hope is that this book will catalyze further interest, research, understanding, and dissemination of knowledge about meditative practices, just as the meeting itself served a similar function in its day. Ultimately, the ongoing development and deployment of mindful awareness and the cultivation of positive emotions, including kindness toward oneself, may well be shown to serve both literally and metaphorically as the mind's own physician, a powerful resource available to all who care to listen deeply to the currents of one's own mind, heart, body, and life. The science is already suggesting on the whole that this may be so, even as, perhaps more importantly, we note the experiences of countless meditation practitioners, who seem to be benefiting in terms of quality of life, health, and well-being from this emerging perspective on the value and practicality of the meditative disciplines.

ACKNOWLEDGMENTS

The editors would like to thank the following:

His Holiness the Dalai Lama for his enduring inspiration and commitment to mutual engagement and inquiry between the contemplative traditions and science, and to rigorous research to expand our understanding of the nature of mind and its potential to adequately address the full scope and dimensionality of human suffering.

Adam Engle for his incomparable leadership of the Mind and Life Institute over the past twenty-five years and, in particular, during the last ten years, when its mission expanded in so many complex and important ways. We owe him an enormous debt of gratitude.

Thupten Jinpa for his remarkable translating skills, his transparent presence, and his boundless commitment to His Holiness.

Judy Martin for her organizational wizardry. Dave Womack for helping secure the photographs for this volume. The entire staff of the Mind and Life Institute for their profound commitment to the mission of Mind and Life and the huge dedication they bring to all aspects of their work, often behind the scenes. To former Mind and Life staff members Nancy A. Mayer, Dave Mayer, Cathy Chen-Ortega, and Sidney Prince for the extraordinary effort, skill, and goodwill they put into organizing the 2005 meeting.

Zara Houshmand for the pleasure of working with her and the benefit of her finely honed intellect and incisive editorial skills, fully tuned to the Mind and Life culture and ethos. Jasmine Star for her excellent, essential, comprehensive, and unrelenting editorial work on the manuscript to bring it into its final form.

The staff of New Harbinger Publications who nurtured the development of this book at every stage with a high degree of professionalism and a seamlessly integrated team so that every base was covered when it needed to be: Catharine Meyers, Jess Beebe, Michele Waters, Adia Colar, Amy Shoup, Heather Garnos, Janice Fitch, Melissa Valentine, and Matt McKay.

We extend our gratitude to all the speakers and panelists for their important contributions to the dialogue, and to all the participants who attended the 2005 meeting. As we noted, the audience constituted a gigantic force at this gathering. Through their presence and their own work, their contributions to the ongoing confluence of these two episte-mological streams are keeping the field vital and endlessly creative.

And finally, we wish to express our deep gratitude to all the people who agreed to be subjects in the various studies that were presented. All of us, and indeed the world, are potential beneficiaries of your engagement in this work. We also acknowledge our deep debt to the animals used in some lines of research.

NOTES

1. G. Synder, *The Practice of the Wild* (San Francisco: North Point Press, 1990), 61. For the meaning of Snyder's use of the word "empty," see J. Kabat-Zinn, *Coming to Our Senses* (New York: Hyperion, 2005), 172–183, and B. A. Wallace and B. Hodel, *Embracing Mind: The Common Ground of Science and Spirituality* (Boston: Shambhala, 2008).

2. F. J. Varela, E. Thompson, and E. Rosch, *The Embodied Mind* (Cambridge, MA: MIT Press, 1991), 14–33; S. Pinker, *How the Mind Works* (New York: Norton, 1997), 147–148.

3. A. Harrington and A. Zajonc, *The Dalai Lama at MIT* (Cambridge, MA: Harvard University Press, 2006), 8.

4. Ibid.

5. D. Goleman, *Destructive Emotions* (New York: Bantam, 2003).

6. A. Harrington and A. Zajonc, *The Dalai Lama at MIT* (Cambridge, MA: Harvard University Press, 2006).

7. J. M. G. Williams and J. Kabat-Zinn, "Mindfulness: Diverse Perspectives on Its Meaning, Origins, and Multiple Applications at the Intersection of Science and Dharma," *Contemporary Buddhism* 12, no. 1 (2011): 1–18.

8. A. Harrington and A. Zajonc, *The Dalai Lama at MIT* (Cambridge, MA: Harvard University Press, 2006), 12.

9. A. K. Anderson, A. Jha, and Z. Segal, "Mindfulness Training and Emotion Regulation: Clinical and Neuroscience Perspectives," special section, *Emotion* 10, no. 1 (2010).

10. S. L. Shapiro (ed.), "Mindfulness," special issue, *Journal of Clinical Psychology* 65, no. 6 (2009).

11. "Recent Developments in Mindfulness-Based Research," special issue, *Journal of Cognitive Psychotherapy* 23, no. 3 (2009).

12. J. Kabat-Zinn and M. Williams (eds.), "Mindfulness: Diverse Perspectives on Its Meaning, Origins, and Multiple Applications at the Intersection of Science and Dharma," special issue, *Contemporary Buddhism* 12, no. 1 (2011).

13. T. Gyatso, HH Dalai Lama, *The Universe in a Single Atom: The Convergence of Science and Spirituality* (New York: Morgan Road Books, 2005).

14. His Holiness is referring to the great Buddhist university at Nalanda in India, which flourished on and off from the fifth to the twelfth century CE. (It was destroyed by invaders three times during that period.)

15. D. Bohm, *Wholeness and the Implicate Order* (London: Routledge and Kegan Paul, 1980).

16. J. Kabat-Zinn, "An Outpatient Program in Behavioral Medicine for Chronic Pain Patients Based on the Practice of Mindfulness Meditation: Theoretical Considerations and Preliminary Results," *General Hospital Psychiatry* 4, no. 1 (1982): 33–47.

17. J. Kabat-Zinn, L. Lipworth, and R. Burney, "The Clinical Use of Mindfulness Meditation for the Self-Regulation of Chronic Pain," *Journal of Behavioral Medicine* 8, no. 2 (1985): 163–190.

18. For example, J. Kabat-Zinn, L. Lipworth, R. Burney, et al., "Four-Year Follow-Up of a Meditation-Based Program for the Self-Regulation of Chronic Pain: Treatment Outcomes and Compliance," *Clinical Journal of Pain* 2, no. 3 (1987): 159–173.

19. As of 2011, the number had risen to 46.

20. R. J. Davidson, J. Kabat-Zinn, J. Schumacher, et al., "Alterations in Brain and Immune Function Produced by Mindfulness Meditation," *Psychosomatic Medicine* 65, no. 4 (2003): 564–570.

21. J. Kabat-Zinn, E. Wheeler, T. Light, et al., "Influence of a Mindfulness-Based Stress Reduction Intervention on Rates of Skin Clearing in

Patients with Moderate to Severe Psoriasis Undergoing Phototherapy (UVB) and Photochemotherapy (PUVA)," *Psychosomatic Medicine* 60, no. 5 (1998): 625–632.

22. Ibid.

23. Ibid.

24. D. Kahneman, "Objective Happiness," in *Well-Being: The Foundations of Hedonic Psychology*, ed. D. Kahneman, E. Diener, and N. Schwarz (New York: Russell Sage Foundation, 1999), 3–25.

25. G. Schlaug, M. Forgeard, L. Zhu, et al., "Training-Induced Neuroplasticity in Young Children," *Annals of the New York Academy of Sciences* (July 2009): 205–208.

26. J. Driemeyer, J. Boyke, C. Gaser, et al., "Changes in Gray Matter Induced by Learning—Revisited," *Public Library of Science One* 3, no. 7 (2008): e2669.

27. T. Y. Zhang and M. J. Meaney, "Epigenetics and the Environmental Regulation of the Genome and Its Function," *Annual Review of Psychology* 6 (2010): 439–466.

28. H. L. Urry, C. M. van Reekum, T. Johnstone, et al., "Amygdala and Ventromedial Prefrontal Cortex Are Inversely Coupled during Regulation of Negative Affect and Predict the Diurnal Pattern of Cortisol Secretion among Older Adults," *Journal of Neuroscience* 26, no. 16 (2006): 4415–4425.

29. Ibid.

30. A. Lutz, L. Greischar, N. B. Rawlings, et al., "Long-Term Meditators Self-Induce High-Amplitude Synchrony during Mental Practice," *Proceedings of the National Academy of Sciences* 101, no. 46 (2004): 16369–16373.

31. R. J. Davidson, J. Kabat-Zinn, J. Schumacher, et al., "Alterations in Brain and Immune Function Produced by Mindfulness Meditation," *Psychosomatic Medicine* 65, no. 4 (2003): 564–570.

32. Ibid.

33. A. Einstein, letter quoted in *New York Times*, March 29, 1972.

34. "Buddhadharma" here means the foundational teachings of the Buddha. Universal dharma is the same understanding but framed in a non-Buddhist, more global context and language.

35. See, for example, K. A. MacLean, E. Ferrer, S. R. Aichele, et al., "Intensive Meditation Training Improves Perceptual Discrimination and Sustained Attention," *Psychological Science* 21, no. 6 (2010): 829–839. For more information and publications from the Shamatha Project see: http://mindbrain.ucdavis.edu/labs/Saron/shamatha-project.

36. W. Singer, "Synchronization of Cortical Activity and Its Putative Role in Information Processing and Learning," *Annual Review of Physiology* 55 (1993): 349–374.

37. W. Singer, "Neuronal Synchrony: A Versatile Code for the Definition of Relations?" *Neuron* 24, no. 1 (1999): 49–65.

38. P. Fries, D. Nikolic, and W. Singer, "The Gamma Cycle," *Trends in Neurosciences* 30, no. 7 (2007): 309–316.

39. W. Singer, "Synchronous Oscillations and Memory Formation," in *Learning and Memory: A Comprehensive Reference*, vol. 1, *Learning Theory and Behavior*, ed. J. Byrne (Oxford: Elsevier, 2008), 721–728.

40. L. Melloni and W. Singer, "Distinct Characteristics of Conscious Experience Are Met by Large-Scale Neuronal Synchronization," in *New Horizons in the Neuroscience of Consciousness*, ed. E. Perry, D. Collerton, F. LeBeau, et al. (Amsterdam: John Benjamins, 2010), 17–28.

41. L. Melloni, C. Molina, M. Pena, et al., "Synchronization of Neural Activity across Cortical Areas Correlates with Conscious Perception," *Journal of Neuroscience* 27, no. 1 (2007): 2858–2865.

42. J. Weiss, "Psychological Factors in Stress and Disease," *Scientific American* 226 (June, 1972): 104–113.

43. R. Sapolsky, "Stress and Cognition," in *The Cognitive Neurosciences* (Cambridge, MA: MIT Press, 2004), 1031–1042.

44. Ibid.

45. C. Gambarana, F. Masi, A. Tagliamonte, et al., "A Chronic Stress That Impairs Reactivity in Rats Also Decreases Dopaminergic

Transmission in the Nucleus Accumbens: A Microdialysis Study," *Journal of Neurochemistry* 72, no. 5 (1999), 2039–2046.

46. A. Vyas, R. Mitra, B. Rao, et al., "Chronic Stress Induces Contrasting Patterns of Dendritic Remodeling in Hippocampal and Amygdaloid Neurons," *Journal of Neuroscience* 22, no. 15 (2002): 6810–6818.

47. J. J. Radley, H. M. Sisti, J. Hao, et al., "Chronic Behavior Stress Induces Apical Dendrite Reorganization in Pyramidal Neurons of the Medial Prefrontal Cortex," *Neuroscience* 125, no. 1 (2004): 1–6.

48. C. D. Fiorillo, P. N. Tobler, and W. Schultz, "Discrete Coding of Reward Probability and Uncertainty by Dopamine Neurons," *Science* 299, no. 5614 (2003): 1898–1902.

49. T. Gyatso, HH Dalai Lama, *The Universe in a Single Atom: The Convergence of Science and Spirituality* (New York: Morgan Road Books, 2005).

50. R. J. Sapolsky and L. J. Share, "A Pacific Culture among Wild Baboons: Its Emergence and Transmission," *Public Library of Science Biology* 2, no. 4 (2004): e106.

51. Rainer Goebel, personal communication.

52. M. Friedman and R. Rosenman, *Type A Behavior and Your Heart* (New York: Knopf, 1974).

53. M. E. Kemeny, L. J. Rosenwasser, R. A. Panettieri, et al., "Placebo Response in Asthma: A Robust and Objective Phenomenon," *Journal of Allergy and Clinical Immunology* 119, no. 6 (2007): 1375–1381.

54. A. Einstein, letter quoted in *New York Times*, March 29, 1972.

55. N. S. Nye, "Kindness," in *Words Under Words: Selected Poems* (Portland, OR: Eighth Mountain Press, 1995), 42.

56. "An Estimated 1 in 10 U.S. Adults Report Depression," Centers for Disease Control and Prevention, www.cdc.gov/Features/ds Depression.

57. "Depression," World Health Organization, Mental Health Programmes and Projects, www.who.int/mental_health/management/depression /definition/en.

58. T. I. Mueller, A. C. Leon, M. B. Keller, et al., "Recurrence after Recovery from Major Depressive Disorder during 15 Years of Observational Follow-Up," *American Journal of Psychiatry* 156, no. 7 (1999): 1000–1006.

59. Ibid.

60. W. James, *The Principles of Psychology* (New York: Henry Holt, 1890), vol. 1, 575.

61. Ibid.

62. S. Lyubomirsky and J. Nolen-Hoeksema, "Effects of Self-Focused Rumination on Negative Thinking and Interpersonal Problem Solving," *Journal of Personality and Social Psychology* 69, no. 1 (1995): 176–190.

63. S. D. Hollon, R. J. DeRubeis, and R. C. Shelton, "Prevention of Relapse Following Cognitive Therapy vs. Medications in Moderate to Severe Depression," *Archives of General Psychiatry* 62, no. 4 (2005): 417–422.

64. Z. V. Segal., M. G. Williams, and J. D. Teasdale, *Mindfulness-Based Cognitive Therapy for Depression: A New Approach to Preventing Relapse* (New York: Guilford Press, 2002).

65. J. D. Teasdale, Z. V. Segal, J. M. Williams, et al., "Prevention of Relapse/Recurrence in Major Depression by Mindfulness-Based Cognitive Therapy," *Journal of Consulting and Clinical Psychology* 68, no. 4 (2000): 615–623.

66. Ibid.

67. S. H. Ma and J. D. Teasdale, "Mindfulness-Based Cognitive Therapy for Depression: Replication and Exploration of Differential Relapse Prevention Effects," *Journal of Consulting and Clinical Psychology* 72, no. 1 (2004): 31–40.

68. J. Piet and E. Hougaard, "The Effect of Mindfulness-Based Cognitive Therapy for Prevention of Relapse in Recurrent Major Depressive Disorder: A Systematic Review and Meta-Analysis," *Clinical Psychology Review* 31, no. 6 (2011): 1032–40.

69. W. James, *The Varieties of Religious Experience* (New York: Longmans, Green, and Co., 1902), 147.

70. H. S. Mayberg, S. K. Brannan, R. K. Mahurin, et al., "Regional Metabolic Effects of Fluoxetine in Major Depression: Serial Changes and Relationship to Clinical Response," *Biological Psychiatry* 48, no. 8 (2000): 830–843.

71. K. Goldapple, Z. Segal, C. Garson, et al., "Modulation of Cortical-Limbic Pathways in Major Depression: Treatment Specific Effects of Cognitive Behavior Therapy Compared to Paroxetine," *Archives of General Psychiatry* 61, no. 1 (2004): 34–41.

72. H. S. Mayberg, A. Lozano, V. Voon, et al., "Deep Brain Stimulation for Treatment-Resistant Depression," *Neuron* 45, no. 5 (2005): 651–660.

73. H. S. Mayberg, M. Liotti, S. K. Brannan, et al., "Reciprocal Limbic-Cortical Function and Negative Mood: Converging PET Findings in Depression and Normal Sadness," *American Journal of Psychiatry* 156, no. 5 (1999): 675–682.

74. K. Goldapple, Z. Segal, C. Garson, et al., "Modulation of Cortical-Limbic Pathways in Major Depression: Treatment-Specific Effects of Cognitive Behavior Therapy Compared to Paroxetine," *Archives of General Psychiatry* 61, no. 1 (2004): 34–41.

75. H. S. Mayberg, "Limbic-Cortical Dysregulation: A Proposed Model of Depression," *Journal of Neuropsychiatry and Clinical Neurosciences* 9, no. 3 (1997): 471–481.

76. H. S. Mayberg, A. Lozano, V. Voon, et al., "Deep Brain Stimulation for Treatment-Resistant Depression," *Neuron* 45, no. 5 (2005): 651–660.

77. J. D. Teasdale, Z. V. Segal, J. M. G. Williams, et al., "Prevention of Relapse/Recurrence in Major Depression by Mindfulness-Based Cognitive Therapy," *Journal of Consulting and Clinical Psychology* 68, no. 4 (2000): 615–623; and S. H. Ma and J. D. Teasdale, "Mindfulness-Based Cognitive Therapy for Depression: Replication and Exploration of Differential Relapse Prevention Effects," *Journal of Consulting and Clinical Psychology* 72, no. 1 (2004), 31–40. Also see J. Piet and E. Hougaard, "The Effect of Mindfulness-Based Cognitive Therapy for Prevention of Relapse in Recurrent Major Depressive Disorder: A

Systematic Review and Meta-Analysis," *Clinical Psychology Review* (in press) for a recent meta-analytic review of all available studies.

78. W. Kuyken, E. Watkins, E. Holden, et al., "How Does Mindfulness-Based Cognitive Therapy Work?" *Behaviour Research and Therapy* 48, no. 1 (2010): 1105–1112.

79. W. James and J. McDermott, *The Writings of William James: A Comprehensive Edition* (Chicago: University of Chicago Press, 1977), 6–8.

80. American Psychiatric Association, *Diagnostic and Statistical Manual of Mental Disorders* (Washington, DC: American Psychiatric Association, 2000).

81. H. S. Mayberg, "Modulating Dysfunctional Limbic-Cortical Circuits in Depression: Towards Development of Brain-Based Algorithms for Diagnosis and Optimised Treatment," *British Medical Bulletin* 65, no. 1 (2003): 193–207.

82. P. Kramer, *Listening to Prozac: The Landmark Book about Antidepressants and the Remaking of the Self* (New York: Viking Penguin, 1993).

83. T. Gyatso, HH Dalai Lama, *The Art of Happiness* (New York: Riverhead Books, 2009), 13.

84. T. Gyatso, HH Dalai Lama, *Ethics for the New Millennium* (New York: Riverhead Books, 2009).

85. N. Birbaumer, N. Ghanayim, T. Hinterberger, et al., "A Spelling Device for the Paralysed," *Nature* 398, no. 6725 (1999): 297–298.

86. S. Yusuf, S. Hawken, S. Ounpuu, et al., "Effect of Potentially Modifiable Risk Factors Associated with Myocardial Infarction in 52 Countries (the INTERHEART study): Case-Control Study," *Lancet* 364, no. 9438 (2004): 937–952.

87. V. Papademetriou, J. S. Gottdiener, W. J. Kop, et al., "Transient Coronary Occlusion with Mental Stress," *American Heart Journal* 132, no. 6 (1996): 1299–1301.

88. M. M. Burg, A. Vashist, and R. Soufer, "Mental Stress Ischemia: Present Status and Future Goals," *Journal of Nuclear Cardiology* 12, no. 5 (2005): 523–529.

89. P. G. Kaufmann, R. P. McMahon, L. C. Becker, et al., "The Psychophysiological Investigations of Myocardial Ischemia (PIMI) Study: Objective, Methods, and Variability of Measures," *Psychosomatic Medicine* 60, no. 1 (1998): 56–63.

90. J. K. Kiecolt-Glaser, R. Glaser, S. Gravenstein, et al., "Chronic Stress Alters the Immune Response to Influenza Vaccine in Older Adults," *Proceedings of the National Academy of Sciences* 93, no. 7 (1996): 3043–3407.

91. R. Glaser, J. K. Kiecolt-Glaser, W. B. Malarkey, et al., "The Influence of Psychological Stress on the Immune Response to Vaccines," *Annals of the New York Academy of Sciences* 840 (May 1998): 649–655.

92. R. Glaser, J. K. Kiecolt-Glaser, R. H. Bonneau, et al., "Stress-Induced Modulation of the Immune Response to Recombinant Hepatitis B Vaccine," *Psychosomatic Medicine* 54, no. 1 (1992): 22–29.

93. R. Glaser, J. Sheridan, J. Malarkey, et al., "Chronic Stress Modulates the Immune Response to a Pneumococcal Pneumonia Vaccine," *Psychosomatic Medicine* 62, no. 6 (2000): 804–807.

94. R. J. Davidson, J. Kabat-Zinn, J. Schumacher, et al., "Alterations in Brain and Immune Function Produced by Mindfulness Meditation," *Psychosomatic Medicine* 65, no. 4 (2003): 564–570.

95. R. J. Tseng, D. A. Padgett, F. S. Dhabhar, et al., "Stress-Induced Modulation of NK Activity during Influenza Viral Infection: Role of Glucocorticoids and Opioids," *Brain, Behavior, and Immunity* 19, no. 2 (2005): 153–164.

96. M. T. Bailey, H. Engler, N. D. Powell, et al., "Repeated Social Defeat Increases the Bactericidal Activity of Splenic Macrophages through a Toll-like Receptor-Dependent Pathway," *American Journal of Physiology: Regulatory, Integrative, and Comparative Physiology* 293, no. 3 (2007): 1180–1190.

97. T. Gyatso, HH Dalai Lama, *The Universe in a Single Atom: The Convergence of Science and Spirituality* (New York: Morgan Road Books, 2005).

98. D. Boorstin, *The Discoverers* (New York: Random House Books, 1983).

99. W. James, *A Pluralistic Universe* (Cambridge, MA: Harvard University Press, 1977), 142.

100. W. Wordsworth, "Prelude," in *The Poetical Works of William Wordsworth*, ed. T. Hutchinson (London: Oxford University Press, 1910), 637.

101. A. Chiesa, R. Calati, and A. Serretti, "Does Mindfulness Training Improve Cognitive Abilities? A Systematic Review of Neuropsychological Findings," *Clinical Psychology Review* 31, no. 3 (2010): 449–464; T. Krisanaprakornkit, C. Ngamjarus, C. Witoonchart, et al., "Meditation Therapies for Attention-Deficit/ Hyperactivity Disorder (ADHD)," *Cochrane Database of Systematic Reviews* 6 (June 16, 2010): CD006507; A. Chiesa and A. Serretti, "A Systematic Review of Neurobiological and Clinical Features of Mindfulness Meditations," *Psychological Medicine* 40, no. 8 (2010): 1239–1252; A. Zgierska, D. Rabago, N. Chawla, et al., "Mindfulness Meditation for Substance Use Disorders: A Systematic Review," *Substance Abuse* 30, no. 4 (2009): 266–294; D. S. Black, J. Milam, and S. Sussman, "Sitting-Meditation Interventions among Youth: A Review of Treatment Efficacy," *Pediatrics* 124, no. 3 (2009): e532–541; K. Rubia, "The Neurobiology of Meditation and Its Clinical Effectiveness in Psychiatric Disorders," *Biological Psychology* 82, no. 1 (2009): 1–11; A. Lutz, J. A. Brefczynski-Lewis, T. Johnstone, et al., "Regulation of the Neural Circuitry of Emotion by Compassion Meditation: Effects of Expertise," *Public Library of Science One* 3, no. 3 (2008): e1897; A. Lutz, H. A. Slagter, J. Dunne, et al., "Attention Regulation and Monitoring in Meditation," *Trends in Cognitive Sciences* 12, no. 4 (2008): 163–169; B. R. Cahn and J. Polich, "Meditation States and Traits: EEG, ERP, and Neuroimaging Studies," *Psychological Bulletin* 132, no. 2 (2006): 180–211; and T. Krisanaprakornkit, W. Krisanaprakornkit, N. Piyavhatkul, et al., "Meditation Therapy for Anxiety Disorders," *Cochrane Database of Systematic Reviews* 1 (January 25, 2006): CD004998.

102. H. A. Slagter, A. Lutz, L. L. Greischar, et al., "Mental Training Affects Distribution of Limited Brain Resources," *Public Library of Science Biology* 5, no. 6 (2007): e138.

103. A. Lutz, H. Slagter, N. Rawling, et al., "Mental Training Enhances Attentional Stability: Neural and Behavioral Evidence," *Journal of Neuroscience* 29, no. 42 (2009): 13418–13427.

104. K. A. MacLean, E. Ferrer, S. R. Aichele, et al., "Intensive Meditation Training Improves Perceptual Discrimination and Sustained Attention," *Psychological Science* 21, no. 6 (2010): 829–839.

105. F. Zeidan, S. K. Johnson, B. J. Diamond, et al., "Mindfulness Meditation Improves Cognition: Evidence of Brief Mental Training," *Consciousness and Cognition* 19, no. 2 (2010): 597–605.

106. A. Wallace, *The Attention Revolution: Unlocking the Power of the Focused Mind* (Boston: Wisdom Publications, 2006).

107. M. Kozhevnikov, O. Louchakova, Z. Josipovic, et al., "The Enhancement of Visuospatial Processing Efficiency through Buddhist Deity Meditation," *Psychological Science* 20, no. 5 (2009): 645–653.

108. J. A. Grant, J. Courtemanche, E. G. Duerden, et al., "Cortical Thickness and Pain Sensitivity in Zen Meditators," *Emotion* 10, no. (2010): 43–53.

109. J. Kabat-Zinn, "An Outpatient Program in Behavioral Medicine for Chronic Pain Patients Based on the Practice of Mindfulness Meditation: Theoretical Considerations and Preliminary Results," *General Hospital Psychiatry* 4, no. 1 (1982): 33–47.

110. A. S. Farb, Z. V. Segal, H. Mayberg, et al., "Attending to the Present: Mindfulness Meditation Reveals Distinct Neural Modes of Self-Reference," *Social Cognitive and Affective Neuroscience* 2, no. 4 (2007): 313–322.

111. M. E. Raichle, A. M. MacLeod, A. Z. Snyder, et al., "A Default Mode of Brain Function," *Proceedings of the National Academy of Sciences* 98, no. 2 (2001): 676–682.

112. M. F. Mason, M. I. Norton, J. D. Van Horn, et al., "Wandering Minds: The Default Network and Stimulus-Independent Thought," *Science* 315, no. 5810 (2007): 393–395.

113. J. M. G. Williams, "Mindfulness, Depression, and Modes of Mind," *Cognitive Therapy and Research* 32, no. 6 (2008): 721–733; J. Kabat-Zinn, *Full Catastrophe Living* (New York: Dell, 1990), 96–97; and J.

Kabat-Zinn, *Wherever You Go, There You Are* (New York: Hyperion, 1994), 14.

114. N. A. Farb, A. K. Anderson, H. Mayberg, et al., "Minding One's Emotions: Mindfulness Training Alters the Neural Expression of Sadness," *Emotion* 10, no. 1 (2010): 25–33.

115. C. E. Kerr, S. R. Jones, Q. Wan, et al., "Effects of Mindfulness Meditation Training on Anticipatory Alpha Modulation in Primary Somatosensory Cortex," *Brain Research Bulletin* 85, no. 3–4 (2011): 96–103.

116. B. K. Hölzel, J. Carmody, M. Vangel, et al., "Mindfulness Practice Leads to Increases in Regional Brain Gray Matter Density," *Psychiatry Research* 191, no. 1 (2011): 36–43.

117. B. K. Hölzel, J. Carmody, K. C. Evans, et al., "Stress Reduction Correlates with Structural Changes in the Amygdala," *Social Cognitive and Affective Neuroscience* 5, no. 1 (2010): 11–17.

118. B. Ditto, M. Eclache, and N. Goldman, "Short-Term Autonomic and Cardiovascular Effects of Mindfulness Body Scan Meditation," *Annals of Behavioral Medicine* 32, no. 3 (2006): 227–234.

119. T. L. Jacobs, E. S. Epel, J. Lin, et al., "Intensive Meditation Training, Immune Cell Telomerase Activity, and Psychological Mediators," *Psychoneuroendocrinology* 36, no. 5 (2010): 664–681.

120. E. S. Epel, E. H. Blackburn, J. Lin, et al., "Accelerated Telomere Shortening in Response to Life Stress," *Proceedings of the National Academy of Sciences* 101, no. 49 (2004): 17312–17315.

121. H. D. Critchley, S. Wiens, P. Rotshtein, et al., "Neural Systems Supporting Interoceptive Awareness," *Nature Neuroscience* 7, no. 2 (2004): 189–195.

122. S. S. Khalsa, D. Rudrauf, A. R. Damasio, et al., "Interoceptive Awareness in Experienced Meditators," *Psychophysiology* 45, no. 4 (2008): 671–677.

123. For a detailed description of this practice, see A. Lutz, H. A. Slagter, J. Dunne, et al., "Attention Regulation and Monitoring in Meditation," *Trends in Cognitive Sciences* 12, no. 4 (2008): 163–169.

124. National Institute for Clinical Excellence, *Depression: Management of Depression in Primary and Secondary Care*, National Clinical Practice Guidelines, no. 23 (London: HMSO, 2004; updated 2009).

125. J. D. Teasdale, Z. V. Segal, J. M. G. Williams, et al., "Prevention of Relapse/Recurrence in Major Depression by Mindfulness-Based Cognitive Therapy," *Journal of Consulting and Clinical Psychology* 68, no. 4 (2000): 615–623; and Z. V. Segal, J. M. G. Williams, and J. D. Teasdale, *Mindfulness-Based Cognitive Therapy for Depression: A New Approach to Preventing Relapse* (New York: Guilford Press, 2002).

126. Z. V. Segal, P. Bieling, T. Young, et al., "Antidepressant Monotherapy vs. Sequential Pharmacotherapy and Mindfulness-Based Cognitive Therapy, or Placebo, for Relapse Prophylaxis in Recurrent Depression," *Archives of General Psychiatry* 67, no. 12 (2010): 1256–1264.

127. P. R. Goldin and J. J. Gross, "Effects of Mindfulness-Based Stress Reduction (MBSR) on Emotion Regulation in Social Anxiety Disorder," *Emotion* 10, no. 1 (2010): 83–91.

128. S. Bowen, N. Chawla, S. E. Collins, et al., "Mindfulness-Based Relapse Prevention for Substance Use Disorders: A Pilot Efficacy Trial," *Substance Abuse* 30, no. 4 (2009): 295–305.

129. K. Witkiewitz and S. Bowen, "Depression, Craving, and Substance Use Following a Randomized Trial of Mindfulness-Based Relapse Prevention," *Journal of Consulting and Clinical Psychology* 78, no. 3 (2010): 362–374.

130. J. A. Brewer, S. Mallik, T. A. Babuscio, et al., "Mindfulness Training for Smoking Cessation: Results from a Randomized Controlled Trial," *Drug and Alcohol Dependence* (June 30, 2011): epub ahead of print.

131. M. B. Ospina, T. K. Bond, M. Karkhaneh, et al., *Meditation Practices for Health: State of the Research*, Evidence Report/Technology Assessment 155 (Rockville, MD: Agency for Healthcare Research and Quality, 2007), v.

132. D. MacCoon, Z. Imel, M. Rosenkranz, et al., "The Validation of a Bona Fide Control Intervention for Mindfulness-Based Stress Reduction (MBSR)," under review.

133. See P. Grossman and N. T. Van Dam, "Mindfulness, by Any Other Name . . . : Trials and Tribulations of *Satî* in Western Psychology and Science," *Contemporary Buddhism* 12, no. 1 (2011): 219–240; and R. A. Baer, "Measuring Mindfulness," *Contemporary Buddhism* 12, no. 1 (2011): 241–262.

134. See, for example, M. A. Rosenkranz, W. W. Busse, T. Johnstone, et al., "Neural Circuitry Underlying the Interaction between Emotion and Asthma Symptom Exacerbation," *Proceedings of the National Academy of Sciences* 102, no. 37 (2005): 13319–13324.

135. D. S. Black, J. Milam, and S. Sussman, "Sitting-Meditation Interventions among Youth: A Review of Treatment Efficacy," *Pediatrics* 124, no. 3 (2009): e532–541.

136. L. Zylowska, D. L. Ackerman, M. H. Yang, et al., "Mindfulness Meditation Training in Adults and Adolescents with ADHD: A Feasibility Study," *Attention Disorders* 11, no. 6 (2008): 737–746.

137. A. Miniño, "Mortality among Teenagers Aged 12–19 Years: United States, 1999–2006," *National Center for Health Statistics Data Brief* 37 (May 2010): 1–8.

138. T. Y. Zhang and M. J. Meaney, "Epigenetics and the Environmental Regulation of the Genome and Its Function," *Annual Review of Psychology* 6 (2010): 439–466.

139. J. A. Dusek, H. H. Out, A. L. Wohlhueter, et al., "Genomic Counter-Stress Changes Induced by the Relaxation Response," *Public Library of Science One* 3, no. 7 (2008): e2576.

140. T. Y. Zhang and M. J. Meaney, "Epigenetics and the Environmental Regulation of the Genome and Its Function," *Annual Review of Psychology* 6 (2010): 439–466.

141. O. Sporns, G. Tononi, and R. Kötter, "The Human Connectome: A Structural Description of the Human Brain," *Public Library of Science Computational Biology* 1, no. 4 (2005): e42.

CONTRIBUTORS

Tenzin Gyatso, the fourteenth Dalai Lama, is the leader of Tibetan Buddhism, the head of the Tibetan government in exile, and a spiritual leader revered worldwide. He was born on July 6, 1935, in a small village called Taktser in northeastern Tibet. Born to a peasant family, he was recognized at the age of two, in accordance with Tibetan tradition, as the reincarnation of his predecessor, the thirteenth Dalai Lama. The Dalai Lamas are manifestations of the Buddha of Compassion, who choose to reincarnate for the purpose of serving human beings. Winner of the Nobel Peace Prize in 1989, he is universally respected as a spokesperson for the compassionate and peaceful resolution of human conflict.

He has traveled extensively, speaking on subjects including universal responsibility, love, compassion, and kindness. Less well-known is his intense personal interest in the sciences. He has said that if he were not a monk, he would have liked to be an engineer. As a youth in Lhasa, it was he who was called on to fix broken machinery in the Potola Palace, be it a clock or a car. He has a vigorous interest in learning the newest developments in science and brings to bear both a voice for the humanistic implications of the findings and a high degree of intuitive methodological sophistication.

Ajahn Amaro is abbot of Amaravati Buddhist Monastery in England and formerly co-abbot of Abhayagiri Buddhist Monastery in Northern California. He received a BSc with honors from London University in psychology and physiology in 1977. In 1978 he took up residence in a forest meditation monastery in the lineage of Ven. Ajahn Chah in northeast Thailand. He returned to England in 1979 to join Ven. Ajahn Sumedho at a newly founded forest monastery in Sussex. In 1983 he journeyed 830 miles on foot to a branch monastery in Northumberland. In 1985 he went to Amaravati Buddhist Monastery and helped with teaching and administration for ten years, serving as vice-abbot for the last two years. In 1990 he started teaching in the United States a few months each year. In 1996 he founded Abhayagiri Monastery, in Mendocino County, California, and was based there until 2010, when he was invited to return to England and take up the position of abbot of Amaravati Monastery.

The main focus of his life is practicing as a forest monk and teaching and training others in that same tradition. He has authored eight books, including *Finding the Missing Peace* (2011), a handbook on Buddhist meditation; *Rugged Interdependency* (2007), commentaries on Buddhist life in the United States; and *Small Boat, Great Mountain: Theravadan Reflections on the Natural Great Perfection* (2003). In addition, he has written numerous articles and coauthored, edited, or contributed to several books, including *The Island: An Anthology of the Buddha's Teachings on Nibbana* (2009); *The Sound of Silence: The Selected Teachings of Ajahn Sumedho* (2007); *Food for the Heart: The Collected Teachings of Ajahn Chah* (2002); *Broad View, Boundless Heart* (2001); and *Dhamma and the Real World* (2000). A number of his books are available online at no charge at www.amaravati.org and at www.abhayagiri.org.

Roshi Jan Chozen Bays is a pediatrician specializing in the evaluation of children for possible abuse and neglect. After graduating from Swarthmore College, she received medical training at the University of California, San Diego. For ten years she served as medical director of the Child Abuse Response and Evaluation Services at Legacy Children's Hospital in Portland, Oregon, where over one thousand children and families are seen each year for concerns of abuse and neglect. She has written a number of articles for medical journals and book chapters on aspects of child abuse, including substance abuse and child abuse, child abuse by poisoning, and conditions mistaken for child abuse.

Jan Chozen Bays has studied and practiced Zen Buddhism since 1973. She was ordained as a Zen priest under Taizan Maezumi Roshi and given authorization to teach in 1983. With her husband, Hogen Bays, she teaches at Zen Community of Oregon and Great Vow Zen Monastery, a residential center for intensive Zen training in Clatskanie, Oregon. She has published articles about Zen in *Tricycle* and *Buddhadharma* magazines. She is the author of *How to Train a Wild Elephant and Other Adventures in Mindfulness*

(2011); *Mindful Eating: Rediscovering a Healthy and Joyful Relationship with Food* (2009); and *Jizo Bodhisattva: Guardian of Children, Women, and Other Voyagers* (2003).

Richard J. Davidson is the director of the Laboratory for Affective Neuroscience, the Waisman Laboratory for Functional Brain Imaging and Behavior, and the Center for Investigating Healthy Minds at the University of Wisconsin at Madison. He was educated at New York University and Harvard University, where he received respectively his BA and PhD in psychology. Over the course of his research career, he has focused on the relationship between brain and emotion. He is currently the William James Professor and Vilas Research Professor of Psychology and Psychiatry at the University of Wisconsin. He is coauthor or editor of thirteen books, including *The Handbook of Affective Sciences* (2009), *Visions of Compassion: Western Scientists and Tibetan Buddhists Examine Human Nature* (2003), and *The Emotional Life of Your Brain* (2012).

Dr. Davidson has also written more than 250 journal articles and book chapters. He is the recipient of numerous awards for his work, including the Research Scientist Award from the National Institute of Mental Health, the Distinguished Scientific Contribution Award from the American Psychological Association, and election to the American Academy of Arts and Sciences. He was a member of the Board of Scientific Counselors of the National Institute of Mental Health. In 1992, as a follow-up from previous Mind and Life meetings, he was a member of a scientific team doing neuroscientific investigations of exceptional mental abilities in advanced Tibetan monks.

John J. DeGioia became the forty-eighth president of Georgetown University on July 1, 2001. He has served the university as both a senior administrator and a faculty member since 1979. Georgetown University is a distinctive educational institution, rooted in the Catholic faith and Jesuit tradition, and therefore committed to spiritual inquiry, engaged in the public sphere, and invigorated by religious and cultural pluralism. As the first lay president of a Jesuit university, Dr. DeGioia places special emphasis on sustaining and strengthening Georgetown's Catholic and Jesuit identity and its responsibility to serve as a voice and an instrument for justice. He is a member of the Order of Malta, a lay religious order of the Roman Catholic Church dedicated to serving the sick and the poor. Dr. DeGioia has been a strong advocate for interreligious dialogue.

To prepare young people for leadership roles in the global community, Dr. DeGioia has expanded opportunities for both interreligious and intercultural dialogue, welcomed world leaders to campus, and convened international conferences to address challenging issues. He is a member of the U.S. National Commission for UNESCO and chair of its Education Committee, and he represents Georgetown at the World Economic Forum and on the Council on Foreign Relations. Dr. DeGioia remains a professorial lecturer in the Department of Philosophy and recently taught Ethics and Global Development. He earned a bachelor's degree in English from Georgetown University in 1979 and his PhD in philosophy from the University in 1995.

Adam Engle is a lawyer, businessman, and entrepreneur who has divided his professional life between the for-profit and nonprofit sectors. Mr. Engle received his JD degree from Harvard Law School and his MBA from Stanford Graduate School of Business. In the for-profit sector, he began his career as a lawyer, practicing for ten years in Beverly Hills, Albuquerque, Santa Barbara, and Tehran. After leaving the practice of law, he formed an investment management firm, focusing on global portfolio management on behalf of individual clients. He also started several business ventures in the United States and Australia.

Mr. Engle began working with various groups in the nonprofit sector in 1970. He first came in contact with the Tibetan community in 1974 and has been working with the community since then. Along with Francisco Varela and the Dalai Lama, he cofounded the Mind and Life Dialogues in 1987. He formed the Mind and Life Institute in 1990, and has been its chair and CEO since then. In 1993, he founded the Colorado Friends of Tibet, a statewide Tibetan support group based in Boulder. He also founded a speakers' series at the Stanford Business School entitled Integrity and Compassion in Business. He was a founding member of the Social Venture Network.

Roshi Joan Halifax, is a Buddhist teacher, anthropologist, author, and social activist. She has worked with dying people since 1970 and is a pioneer in the education of clinicians in the end-of-life care field. She is founding abbot and head teacher of Upaya Zen Center and Institute in

Santa Fe, New Mexico. She founded the Ojai Foundation, the Project on Being with Dying, the Upaya Prison Project, and the National Network of Contemplative Prison Programs and is a cofounder of the Zen Peacemaker Order. Her various academic honors have included a National Science Foundation fellowship in Visual Anthropology, honorary research fellow at Harvard University's Peabody Museum, Rockefeller Chair at the California Institute of Integral Studies, and the Harold C. Wit Chair at Harvard Divinity School.

Her books include *Being with Dying: Cultivating Compassion and Fearlessness in the Presence of Death* (2008); *Being with Dying: Compassionate End-of-Life Care Training Guide* (with Barbara Dossey and Cynda Rushton, 2007); *The Fruitful Darkness: A Journey through Buddhist Practice and Tribal Wisdom* (2004); *A Buddhist Life in America: Simplicity in the Complex* (1998); *Shamanic Voices* (1991); *Shaman: The Wounded Healer* (1988); and *The Human Encounter with Death* (with Stanislav Grof, 1978). Among many sound recordings of her lectures, she has done a six CD series for Sounds True entitled *Being with Dying*.

She is cochair of the Lindisfarne Fellows and a board member and fellow of the Mind and Life Institute. She has practiced Buddhism since 1965 and received refuge vows in 1976 from Zen master Seung Sahn. In 1980 she was ordained as a teacher in the Kwan Um School of Zen. In 1990 she received the lamp transmission from Zen master Thich Nhat Hanh. In 1997 she was ordained as a Soto priest by Roshi Bernard Glassman. In 1999 she received dharma transmission and inka from Roshi Glassman.

Thupten Jinpa was educated in the classical Tibetan monastic academia and received the highest academic degree of Geshe Lharam (equivalent to a doctorate in divinity). Jinpa also holds a BA in philosophy and a PhD in religious studies, both from the University of Cambridge, United Kingdom, where he also worked as a research fellow for three years. Since 1985, he has been the principal translator to the Dalai Lama, accompanying him to the United States, Canada, and Europe. He has translated and edited many books by the Dalai Lama, including the *New York Times* best seller *Ethics for the New Millennium* (2001).

His published works also include scholarly articles on various aspects of Tibetan culture, Buddhism, and philosophy, including the entries on Tibetan philosophy for *Encyclopedia of Asian Philosophy* (2001). His latest works include *Self, Reality, and Reason in Tibetan Philosophy: Tsongkhapa's*

Quest for the Middle Way (2002) and the translations *Mind Training: The Great Collection* (2006) and *Songs of Spiritual Experience: Tibetan Poems of Awakening and Insight*, with Jas Elsner (2000). He is on the advisory board of various educational and cultural organizations in North America, Europe, and India and is also the book reviews editor for *Contemporary Buddhism*, a biannual interdisciplinary journal exploring the interface between Buddhism and modern society. He is currently the president and the editor in chief of the Institute of Tibetan Classics, a nonprofit educational organization dedicated to translating key Tibetan classics into contemporary languages.

Jon Kabat-Zinn is founder of mindfulness-based stress reduction (MBSR) and of the Center for Mindfulness in Medicine, Health Care, and Society and professor of medicine emeritus at the University of Massachusetts Medical School. His books include *Mindfulness for Beginners* (2012); *Coming to Our Senses* (2005); *Wherever You Go, There You Are* (1994); and *Full Catastrophe Living* (1990). He has also coauthored several books, including, with Mark Williams, John Teasdale, and Zindel Segal, *The Mindful Way through Depression* (2007); and with his wife, Myla, *Everyday Blessings* (1997). His books have been translated into over thirty languages. He received his PhD in molecular biology from MIT in 1971 with Nobel Laureate Salvador Luria.

He is the author of a series of research papers on the clinical applications of mindfulness. He has trained groups of judges, business leaders, lawyers, Catholic priests, and Olympic athletes in mindfulness and directed multiyear programs in the inner city of Worcester and in the Massachusetts state prison system. He lectures and conducts workshops and training retreat programs in MBSR for health professionals around the world. He is the recipient of awards from educational and medical centers for his work, including the 2008 Mind and Brain Prize from the Center for Cognitive Science, University of Turin, Italy. He is a founding fellow of the Fetzer Institute, a fellow of the Society of Behavioral Medicine, and the founding convener of the Consortium of Academic Health Centers for Integrative Medicine. He is a board member of the Mind and Life Institute and was a presenter at Mind and Life III.

Father Thomas Keating received his BA from Fordham University and, in January 1944, entered the Cistercian Order in Valley Falls, Rhode

Island. He was elected abbot of St. Joseph's Abbey, Spencer, Massachusetts, in 1961. He is one of the architects of the centering prayer movement, begun in Spencer Abbey in 1975, a contemporary form of the Christian contemplative tradition. In 1984 he founded Contemplative Outreach, Ltd., now an international ecumenical organization that teaches centering prayer and the Christian contemplative tradition, and provides a support system for those on the contemplative path through a wide variety of resources, workshops, and retreats.

After retiring as abbot of Spencer in 1981, he moved to Snowmass, Colorado, where he established a program of ten-day intensive retreats in the practice of centering prayer, a contemporary form of the Christian contemplative tradition. He helped found the Snowmass Interreligious Conference in 1982 and is a past president of the Temple of Understanding and of the Monastic Interreligious Dialogue, among other interreligious activities. His books include *Divine Therapy and Addiction: Centering Prayer and the Twelve Steps* (2009); *The Human Condition: Contemplation and Transformation* (1999); *Intimacy with God* (1994); *Invitation to Love: The Way of Christian Contemplation* (1992); and *Open Mind, Open Heart: The Contemplative Dimension of the Gospel* (1986).

Margaret E. Kemeny is professor of psychiatry and the director of the Health Psychology Program at the University of California, San Francisco. After spending her undergraduate years at UC, Berkeley, she received her PhD in health psychology from UCSF and completed a four-year post-doctoral fellowship in immunology/psychoneuroimmunology at UCLA. Dr. Kemeny's research has focused on identifying the links between psychological factors, the immune system, and health and illness. She has made important contributions to our understanding of the ways in which the mind—one's thoughts and feelings—shapes biological responses to stress and trauma.

Over the past twenty years she has investigated the role that specific psychological responses play in predicting changes in hormonal and immunological processes relevant to health. This work has been conducted in patient populations (HIV infection and other immune disorders) as well as in healthy individuals. More recently, she has focused on the inflammatory processes relevant to the course of a variety of diseases. She is particularly interested in psychological responses that can ameliorate the stress response and promote positive neuroimmunologic processes relevant to health. In this context she has examined the placebo response in physical disease as well as the role of expectation in disease course. She has been actively involved in a number of intervention studies that incorporate meditation and contemplative practices to promote emotional and physiological health. Dr. Kemeny has authored or contributed to more than one hundred articles and book chapters in psychological and medical publications.

Jack Kornfield was trained as a Buddhist monk in Thailand, Burma, and India and has taught meditation around the world since 1974. He is one of the main teachers to introduce Theravada Buddhist practice to the West. His work has been focused on integrating Eastern spiritual teachings in a way that is accessible to Western society. He graduated from Dartmouth College in Asian Studies and holds a PhD in clinical psychology from Saybrook University. His doctoral dissertation was one of the first to explore the psychology of mindfulness meditation. Jack is a husband and father, and a founding teacher of two of the largest meditation centers in the West, the Insight Meditation Society and Spirit Rock Meditation Center.

He has published a number of articles on the interface of Eastern and Western psychology. His books include *Bringing Home the Dharma: Awakening Right Where You Are* (2011); *The Wise Heart: A Guide to the Universal Teachings of Buddhist Psychology* (2008); *Living Dharma* (1995); *Buddha's Little Instruction Book* (1994); *A Path with Heart* (1993); *After the Ecstasy, the Laundry* (2000); and *The Art of Forgiveness, Loving-Kindness, and Peace* (2002). He has also coauthored *Seeking the Heart of Wisdom* (1987) and edited *Stories of the Spirit, Stories of the Heart: Parables of the Spiritual Path from Around the World* (1991) and *A Still Forest Pool: The Insight Meditation of Achaan Chah* (1985).

Helen S. Mayberg is professor of psychiatry and neurology at Emory University School of Medicine and the Dorothy C. Fuqua Chair in Psychiatric Neuroimaging and Therapeutics. She received her BA in psychobiology from University of California, Los Angeles, and MD degree from the University of Southern California. Following an internship in internal medicine at the Los Angeles County + USC Medical Center and a residency in neurology at the Neurological Institute of New York at Columbia University's College of Physicians and Surgeons, she completed a postdoctoral fellowship in nuclear medicine at Johns Hopkins University. Dr. Mayberg has held academic positions at Johns Hopkins and the University of Texas Health Science Center at San Antonio and was the first Sandra A. Rotman Chair in Neuropsychiatry at the Rotman Research Institute at the University of Toronto.

The central theme of her research program is the use of functional neuroimaging methods to define critical neural pathways mediating normal and abnormal mood states in health and disease. Converging findings from a series of studies has led to a neural systems model of major depression. This model provides the foundation for ongoing experiments examining mechanisms of standard treatments such as cognitive behavioral therapy and pharmacotherapy, as well as the development of a novel surgical intervention using deep brain stimulation for patients who don't respond to other treatments. In 2004 she moved to Emory University in Atlanta, where her studies have expanded to address neurobiological markers predicting treatment response, relapse, and resistance, as well as vulnerability to depression, with a goal of developing imaging-based algorithms that will discriminate patient subgroups and optimize treatment selection for individual patients.

Edward D. Miller was named CEO of Johns Hopkins Medicine and the thirteenth dean of the Johns Hopkins University School of Medicine in January 1997. He has been responsible for rebuilding and renovation of the medical campus, including two new state-of-the art hospitals, the new Wilmer Building, and a new Medical Education Building, among others that have been completed during his tenure. He directed the implementation of a diversity initiative that places diversity and inclusion as a core fundamental within Johns Hopkins Medicine, and a new curriculum, Genes to Society, and the medical school continues to rank at the top of NIH research funding. He has also implemented initiatives to improve patient safety.

He is a member of the Institute of Medicine and is a fellow of the Royal College of Physicians and the Royal College of Anaesthetists. He has authored or coauthored more than 150 scientific papers, abstracts, and book chapters.

Matthieu Ricard, is a Buddhist monk who lives in Nepal. In 1972, after completing his doctoral thesis in cell genetics at the Pasteur Institute, he began to devote himself to the study of Buddhism in the Himalayas. He is the author of several books, including *Why Meditate? Working with Thoughts and Emotions* (2010); *Happiness: A Guide to Developing Life's Most Important Skill* (2007); *The Quantum and the Lotus* (2004), a dialogue with the astrophysicist Trinh Xuan Thuan; and *The Monk and the Philosopher: A Father and Son Discuss the Meaning of Life* (2000). For four decades, he has been photographing the spiritual masters, landscapes, and people of the Himalayas and is the author-photographer of several albums, including *Bhutan: The Land of Serenity* (2009); *Motionless Journey: From a Hermitage in the Himalayas* (2008); *Tibet: An Inner Journey* (2007); and *Buddhist Himalayas* (2002); and *Journey to Enlightenment* (1996).

He is an active participant in scientific research on the effects of meditation on the brain, working in conjunction with the Mind and Life Institute, and has been the French interpreter for the Dalai Lama since 1989. He is the main coordinator for Karuna-Shechen (karuna-shechen .org), a nonprofit, secular, apolitical organization that has accomplished over one hundred humanitarian projects in Nepal, Tibet, and India, to which he donates all the proceeds of his books and conferences. For more information, see www.matthieuricard.org.

Sharon Salzberg has been a student of meditation since 1971 and has been leading meditation retreats worldwide since 1974. She teaches both intensive awareness practice (vipassana or insight meditation) and the profound cultivation of loving-kindness and compassion (the brahmaviharas).

Sharon's latest book is the *New York Times* best seller *Real Happiness: The Power of Meditation: A 28-Day Program* (2010). She is also the author of *The Force of Kindness* (2010); *The Kindness Handbook* (2008); *Faith: Trusting Your Own Deepest Experience* (2003); *Lovingkindness: The Revolutionary Art of Happiness* (2002); and *A Heart as Wide as the World* (1999); and coauthor with Joseph Goldstein of *Insight Meditation, a Step-by-Step Course on How to Meditate* (audio). She also edited *Voices of Insight* (2001), an anthology of writings by vipassana teachers in the West.

Sharon is cofounder of the Insight Meditation Society in Barre, Massachusetts. She has played a crucial role in bringing Asian meditation practices to the West. The ancient Buddhist practices of vipassana (mindfulness) and metta (loving-kindness) are the foundations of her work. She believes that each of us has a genuine capacity for love, forgiveness, wisdom, and compassion and that meditation awakens these qualities so that we can discover for ourselves the unique happiness that is our birthright. For more information about Sharon, please visit www.sharonsalzberg.com.

Robert Sapolsky is John A. and Cynthia Fry Gunn Professor of Biological Sciences and Neurology and Neurological Sciences at Stanford University, and is a research associate at the Institute of Primate Research, National Museums of Kenya. His work is in three broad areas: how stress and stress hormones damage the nervous system and compromise the ability of neurons to survive neurological insults; the design of gene therapy strategies to protect the nervous system from neurological and psychiatric disorders; and long-standing studies of wild baboons in East Africa, examining the relationships among dominance rank, social behavior, personality, and patterns of stress-related disease. He is the author of more than four hundred technical papers and a number of books for nonscientists, including *Monkeyluv: And Other Essays on Our Lives as Animals* (2005); *A Primate's Memoir: A Neuroscientist's Unconventional Life among the Baboons* (2002); *The Trouble with Testosterone: And Other Essays on the Biology of the Human Predicament* (1998); and *Why Zebras Don't Get Ulcers* (1994).

Zindel Segal, is the Cameron Wilson Chair in Depression Studies and head of the Mood and Anxiety Disorders Program in the Department of Psychiatry at the University of Toronto. He is also head of the Cognitive Behavioural Therapy Clinic at the Centre for Addiction and Mental Health and is a professor in the Department of Psychiatry at the University of Toronto. For more than thirty-five years, Dr. Segal has studied and published widely on psychological treatments for depression, especially the nature of psychological prophylaxis for this recurrent and disabling disorder. His early work helped characterize psychological markers of relapse vulnerability in affective disorder. More recently, he and his colleagues have pioneered the combined use of mindfulness meditation and cognitive therapy as an effective treatment for preventing relapse. Patients who practice mindfulness develop metacognitive awareness of their emotions, which reduces their reactivity to negative affect. Dr. Segal's publications include *Mindfulness-Based Cognitive Therapy for Depression* (2002) and *The Mindful Way through Depression* (2007), a patient guide that outlines this approach.

Bennett M. Shapiro is a consultant in biotechnology. He was previously executive vice president of Worldwide Licensing and External Research for Merck, where he directed Merck's research relationships with the academic and industrial biomedical research community. He joined Merck Research Laboratories in September of 1990 as executive vice president of Basic Research. In this position he was responsible for all of the basic and preclinical research activities at Merck worldwide.

Earlier, he was professor and chairman of the Department of Biochemistry at the University of Washington. He is the author of over 120 papers on the molecular regulation of cellular behavior and the biochemical events that integrate the cascade of cellular activations at fertilization.

Shapiro received his bachelor's degree in chemistry from Dickinson College and his doctor's degree in medicine from Jefferson Medical College. Following an internship in Medicine at the University of Pennsylvania Hospital, he was a research associate at the NIH, then a visiting scientist at the Institut Pasteur in Paris, and then returned to the NIH as chief of the Section on Cellular Differentiation in the Laboratory of Biochemistry prior to joining the University of Washington. Dr. Shapiro has been a Guggenheim Fellow, a Fellow of the Japan Society for the Promotion of Science, and a visiting professor at the University of Nice.

David S. Sheps received his MD from the University of North Carolina (1969), completed his residency in the Department of Medicine at Mount Sinai Hospital (1972), and completed a fellowship in cardiology at Yale University School of Medicine (1974). He earned a master of science degree in public health in epidemiology from the University of North Carolina (1988). Dr. Sheps is a professor of cardiology at Emory University School of Medicine, in Atlanta, Georgia.

Dr. Sheps is a well-recognized expert on the effects of psychological stress in patients with coronary artery disease and mental stress ischemia. He has been principal investigator on numerous grants funded by the NIH, the Health Effects Institute, the U.S. Environmental Protection Agency, and pharmaceutical groups and has focused on behavioral, clinical, and epidemiologic manifestations of disease expression, particularly in coronary artery disease. He was the previous principal investigator of the Women's Health Initiative at the University of North Carolina and has continued his work in that area as the principal investigator of an ancillary study. Dr. Sheps was also a member of the Coordinating Center of the ENRICHD Study, evaluating treatment of depression in patients with coronary artery disease. An ongoing NIH grant, Mindfulness-Based Stress Reduction and Myocardial Ischemia, focuses on treatment of patients with psychological stress–induced ischemia in an attempt to determine whether adverse prognoses can be altered.

John F. Sheridan is professor of immunology and director of the Comprehensive Training in Oral and Craniofacial Sciences program at Ohio State University. He holds the George C. Paffenbarger Alumni Endowed Research Chair and is the associate director of the Institute for Behavioral Medicine Research at Ohio State University. He received a BS degree from Fordham University, and MS and PhD degrees from the Waksman Institute of Microbiology at Rutgers University. He did post-doctoral training in microbiology and immunology at Duke University Medical Center and the Johns Hopkins University School of Medicine.

He is a founding member and past president of the Psychoneuro-immunology Research Society and a fellow of the American Association for the Advancement of Science. His major research interests include neuroendocrine regulation of gene expression in inflammatory and immune responses, stress-induced susceptibility to infectious disease, viral pathogenesis, and host immunity.

Wolf Singer is director at the Max Planck Institute for Brain Research in Frankfurt and founding director of the Frankfurt Institute for Advanced Studies and of the Ernst Strüngmann Institute for Brain Research. He studied medicine at the Universities of Munich and Paris, received his MD from the Ludwig Maximilians University and his PhD from the Technical University in Munich. Until the mid-1980s his research interests were focused on the experience-dependent development of the cerebral cortex and on mechanisms of use-dependent synaptic plasticity. Subsequently, his research concentrated on the binding problem that arises from the distributed organization of the cerebral cortex. The hypothesis forwarded by Professor Singer is that the numerous and widely distributed sub-processes that constitute the basis of cognitive and executive functions are coordinated and bound together by the precise temporal synchronization of oscillatory neuronal activity.

Professor Singer's published works include more than 330 articles in peer-reviewed journals, more than 260 chapters in books, numerous essays on the ethical and philosophical implications of neuroscientific discoveries, and five books. He is the recipient of numerous awards, including the IPSEN Prize for Neuronal Plasticity, the Ernst Jung Prize for Medicine, the

Zülch Prize for Brain Research, the Communicator Prize of the German Research Foundation, and the INNS Hebb Award. He was awarded an honorary doctorate from Oldenburg University and Rutgers University. He is a member of numerous national and international academies, including the Pontifical Academy of Sciences. He has served as president of the European Neuroscience Association, as chairman of the board of directors of the Max Planck Society, and as a member of numerous advisory boards of scientific organizations and editorial boards of journals.

Ralph Snyderman is chancellor emeritus at Duke University and James B. Duke Professor of Medicine in the Duke University School of Medicine. From 1989 to July 2004, he served as chancellor for Health Affairs and dean of the School of Medicine at Duke University. During this period, he oversaw the development of the Duke University Health System, one of the few fully integrated academic health systems in the country, and served as its chief executive officer. The health system not only provides leading-edge care, but also is developing tomorrow's models of health care delivery.

Dr. Snyderman has been a leading proponent of a new approach to health called prospective care. This model envisions each individual receiving a personalized health plan based on his or her own risks and needs. This will give people far more control of and responsibility for their own health as well as opportunities to improve it. Prospective care combines the best in science and technology with humanistic medical practice and relies on integrative medicine to do this.

Dr. Snyderman is the recipient of numerous honors, including the highest award in the field of inflammation research, the Lifetime Achievement Award from the Arthritis Foundation, and the first Bravewell Leadership Award for outstanding achievements in the field of integrative medicine. He is a member of the Institute of Medicine and American Academy of Arts and Sciences, past chair of the Association of American Medical Colleges, and past president of the Association of American Physicians.

Esther M. Sternberg is internationally recognized for her discoveries in brain-immune interactions and the effects of the brain's stress response on health: the science of the mind-body interaction. Dr. Sternberg received her MD degree and trained in rheumatology at McGill University, Montreal, Canada, and served on the faculty at Washington University, St. Louis, Missouri, before joining the National Institutes of Health in

1986. In addition to numerous publications in leading scientific journals, she has edited several textbooks and authored two popular books: the best-selling *Healing Spaces: The Science of Place and Well-Being* (2009) and *The Balance Within: The Science Connecting Health and Emotions* (2000). Dr. Sternberg is a regular contributor to *Science* magazine's "Books et al." section and writes a regular column for the Arthritis Foundation's *Arthritis Today*. Frequently featured in the media, in 2009 she created and hosted a PBS television special, *The Science of Healing*, based on her books.

Dr. Sternberg is currently chief of the Section on Neuroendocrine Immunology and Behavior at the National Institute of Mental Health, director of the Integrative Neural Immune Program, NIMH/NIH, and cochair of the NIH Intramural Program on Research on Women's Health. In recognition of her work, she has received many awards, including the Public Health Service's Superior Service Award, FDA Commissioner's Special Citation, and NIH Director's Challenge Award. She was elected to the American Society for Clinical Investigation, was member of a committee of the National Academy of Sciences Institute of Medicine, testified before Congress, and was an advisor to the World Health Organization. Dr. Sternberg has been an invited lecturer at the Smithsonian Institution (Washington, DC), Nobel Forum (Karolinska Institute, Stockholm), and Royal Society of Medicine (London, UK) and was an invited delegate at *Fortune* magazine's Most Powerful Women Summit and a September 11 panelist at the United Nations, 2008. Dr. Sternberg is one of three hundred women physicians featured in the National Library of Medicine exhibition on women in medicine: "Changing the Face of Medicine." In November 2011 Trinity College, Dublin, will award Dr. Sternberg an Honorary Degree of Doctor in Medicine (Doctorate Honoris Causa). For more information see www.esthersternberg.com.

John Teasdale received his first degree in psychology from the University of Cambridge. Subsequently, he studied for his PhD in abnormal psychology and trained as a clinical psychologist at the Institute of Psychiatry, University of London, where he then taught for a number of years. After working as a National Health Service clinical psychologist in the University Hospital of Wales, he began a thirty-year period of full-time research, supported by the Medical Research Council, first in the Department of Psychiatry, University of Oxford, and subsequently in the MRC Cognition and Brain Sciences Unit, Cambridge.

The continuing focus of his research has been the investigation of basic psychological processes and the application of that understanding to relief from emotional disorders. This involved first the development and evaluation of behavioral therapies for anxiety disorders, then the exploration of cognitive approaches to understanding and treating major depression, and, most recently, the development of mindfulness-based cognitive therapy, a program that is effective in substantially reducing future risk of major depression through an integration of mindfulness training and cognitive approaches.

Dr. Teasdale has published more than one hundred scientific papers and chapters and coauthored three books. He has received a Distinguished Scientist Award from the American Psychological Association and has been elected fellow of both the British Academy and the Academy of Medical Sciences. He is retired and pursuing personal interests in practicing, studying, and teaching meditation and its background.

B. Alan Wallace is president of the Santa Barbara Institute for Consciousness Studies. He trained for many years as a monk in Buddhist monasteries in India and Switzerland. He has taught Buddhist theory and practice in Europe and America since 1976 and has served as interpreter for numerous Tibetan scholars and contemplatives, including the Dalai Lama. After graduating summa cum laude from Amherst College, where he studied physics and the philosophy of science, he earned his MA and PhD in religious studies at Stanford University. He has edited, translated, authored, and contributed to more than forty books on the interface between science and religion and on Tibetan Buddhism, medicine, language, and culture.

His published works include *Meditations of a Buddhist Skeptic: A Manifesto for the Mind Sciences and Contemplative Practice* (2011); *Mind in the Balance: Meditation in Science, Buddhism, and Christianity* (2009); *Embracing Mind: The Common Ground of Science and Spirituality* (2008); *Hidden Dimensions: The Unification of Physics and Consciousness* (2007); *Contemplative Science: Where Buddhism and Neuroscience Converge* (2007); *Buddhism and Science: Breaking New Ground* (2003); *The Taboo of Subjectivity: Toward a New Science of Consciousness* (2000); *The Bridge of Quiescence: Experiencing Buddhist Meditation* (1998); and *Choosing Reality: A Buddhist View of Physics and the Mind* (1996). For more information, consult his website: www.alanwallace.org.

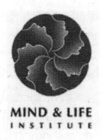

MIND & LIFE
INSTITUTE

ABOUT THE MIND
AND LIFE INSTITUTE

The Mind and Life Institute was cofounded in 1987 by the Dalai Lama, entrepreneur Adam Engle, and neuroscientist Francisco Varela for the purpose of creating rigorous dialogue and research collaboration between modern sciences, the world's living contemplative traditions, philosophy, humanities, and social sciences. We believe this integrated, multidisciplinary research collaboration is the most effective approach to investigating the human mind, developing a more complete understanding of the nature of reality, alleviating suffering, and promoting well-being on the planet.

Over the past two and a half decades, the Mind and Life Institute has become a world leader in cultivating this integrated investigation and developing research fields that explore the effects of contemplative-based practices on the brain, human biology, and behavior.

At the Mind and Life Institute we understand that the world's most serious problems—wars, environmental degradation, poverty, inequality, and social injustice—come from the minds of men and women. In addition, research is showing that mental factors and attitudes contribute to personal illness. We envision a world that fully comprehends the critical importance of training the mind and developing inner resources in ways that alleviate suffering rather than cause suffering, a world in which every-one has access to age-appropriate and culturally appropriate means for accomplishing this inner development.

The mission of the Mind and Life Institute is to:

- Develop the strategy and conceptual framework for a rigor-ous, integrated, multidisciplinary investigation of the mind that combines first- and second-person direct human experi-ence with a modern scientific third-person inquiry

- Develop a global community of scientists and scholars to con-duct this investigation, and global communities of financial partners to provide the material resources to support this research

- Delineate and initiate specific, proof-of-concept research projects that are strategically designed to advance these emerging fields of research

- Communicate research findings to provide a scientific basis for developing and refining practices and programs designed to improve lives and societies, practices that cultivate the human qualities of attention, emotional balance, kindness, compassion, confidence, and happiness

To execute our vision and mission, we have developed a comprehen-sive strategy of integrated initiatives:

- Mind and Life Dialogues with His Holiness the Dalai Lama (23 dialogues since 1987)

- Mind and Life publications, which report on these dialogues (11 books, 5 DVD sets, and 1 online video)

- Mind and Life Summer Research Institute, which helps train scientists and scholars in the emerging fields of contemplative science and contemplative studies (8 institutes serving 1,000 people since 2004)

- Mind and Life Francisco J. Varela Research Awards, which provide pilot research grants to pioneering investigators in contemplative science and contemplative studies (90 research awards totaling $1 million since 2004)

- Mind and Life Humanities and Social Sciences Initiative, which ensures that the emerging fields of contemplative science and contemplative studies are multidisciplinary and integrate first-, second-, and third-person modes of investigation

- Mind and Life Developmental Science Research Network, which investigates how contemplative-based interventions affect human development, with special focus on attention deficit disorders

- Mind and Life Institute Collaborative Coordinator Initiative, which promotes cooperation among the emerging research centers and laboratories in contemplative science and contemplative studies

- International Symposia on Contemplative Studies, an annual networking and information-sharing conference for the emerging fields within contemplative science and contemplative studies

- Publication of papers discussing best practices in contemplative research

To find out more about the Mind and Life Institute, please visit our website at www.mindandlife.org.

The Mind and Life Institute is a nonprofit, tax-exempt 501(c)(3) organization.

7007 Winchester Circle, Suite 100
Boulder, Colorado 80301
303-530-1940

INDEX

evolution of, 186–187, 190; function
and structure changes in, 210–212;
immune system and, 156; increasing
activity in, 93; meditation practice
and, 51–52, 58, 210–212; societies
compared to, 190; synchronized
activity in, 66–67, 69–76

breath, focusing on, 31–32

Buddhism: clinical medicine and,
169–170; cognition in, 193–194;
Eightfold Path of, 29; Four Noble
Truths of, 29, 36; idea of no-self in,
163–164; investigation process in,
22–23, 32; liberation as goal of, 117;
meditation practice in, 31, 33–34,
57, 89; mental health defined in,
124; science of human flourishing
in, 136–144; sensory vs. mental
experience in, 23, 30, 82; suffering
viewed in, 28–29, 30; theory or
worldview of, 139–141

Buddhist psychology, 124–125

C

camera analogy, 32
cardiovascular disease. See heart
disease
Cartesian self, 60
catecholamines, 158
childbed fever, 181
children, meditation for, 219
Christian spiritual tradition, 22,
61–62, 198
chronic vs. acute stress, 37
cigarette smoking, 216
clinical depression, 102–103, 180
clinical research, 214–216
cognitive balance, 142–143
cognitive behavioral therapy, 113–114,
119

cognitive processes: Buddhist view of,
82, 193–194; determining validity
of, 193–194, 199; research on
meditation and, 208–209;
synchronous brain activity and, 70.
See also thoughts
cognitive therapy, 107
community, 91–92, 124
compassion: cultivation of, 165, 166;
forms of, 126; importance of, 201;
long-distance, 191; meditation and,
52–53, 185; wisdom and, 202
component analysis, 119
conative balance, 142
concentration, 161
concluding dialogue, 192–205
conduct, 141
confinement stress, 158
Contemplative Outreach, 198
contemplative traditions: Christian
meditation and, 61–62; convergence
of science and, 2–3, 26, 57; illusion
of knowledge in, 199–200; Mind
and Life XIII participants from,
9–10. See also meditation
Contemporary Buddhism journal, 13
control, sense of, 78, 81, 91
control/comparison groups, 216
Copernicus, Nicolaus, 140
coronary artery disease. See heart
disease
cortex, 49–50
cortisol, 50–51
culture: post-traumatic stress and,
90–91; Western vs. Eastern
worldview and, 187–188

D

Dalai Lama: biographical sketch of,
239; Biological Substrates of
Meditation panel participation, 82,